CONTENTS

This book would not have been possible without the support of many people. First, I owe most of what I know about Type 1 diabetes to Eric's diabetes team, consisting of my coauthors, pediatric endocrinologist Jerrold S. Olshan, MD, and Maryann Waterman, PNP, FNP, CDE, as well as diabetes educators Jennessa Feeney, BSN, RN, CDE, Mary Zamarripa, RD, CDE, and Eric's pediatrician, James Foster, MD. Many thanks are due also to the TuDiabetes. org community for supporting me when I was overwhelmed in the early days after the diagnosis. I would like to thank Jeff McKinnon, Richard Bilodeau, and Betsy Peters for their understanding during the difficult weeks and months after Eric's diagnosis, and my coworkers Marcella Sweet-Demetriou, Amy Amoroso, and Joan Everett for their unfailing support. Thanks are due to Rachel Simpson and Pam Ryder for reading the manuscript and giving an "insider's" perspective on it, and a special nod of gratitude goes to Michelle Jolin and Katie Lovejoy, who were willing to undertake diabetes care education so that my son could continue to attend daycare—I doubt they'll ever truly appreciate what a huge help it has been to know that Eric is in their capable hands while I'm working. Thanks also to Chris Davis, Laura Burns, Kathy Richardson, Brenda Corbett, Daniel Stone, and the rest of the crew at Jones & Bartlett Learning for making this book a reality. And finally, I give my deepest appreciation to my family, who kept the ship afloat while I worked on this project: Eric's daddy, Mark Hamblin; my stepchildren Thomas and Marcayla Hamblin; my mother Nancy Platt; and last but not least, my sons Nathaniel and Eric, who brighten my days more than enough to make up for the occasional insomnia they cause.

Elizabeth Platt

There are a number of good books out there for the parents of children with Type 1 diabetes. Why write another one?

The answer lies in an article published in 2009 in *The Lancet*. The article reviewed European registers of Type 1 diabetes incidence and concluded that while Type 1 diabetes is rising in all age groups, the group with the fastest rise is the 0–5 age group—preschoolers, toddlers, and infants.

When I brought my 18-month-old son, Eric, to the emergency department at Maine Medical Center after his pediatrician had diagnosed his diabetes, I knew instinctively that it was unusual for a child that young to get a diabetes diagnosis. Dr. Olshan, who was the pediatric endocrinologist on call that day, met us at the door of the emergency department, and he quickly confirmed that feeling: "We don't get very many *this* young," he said, adding, "…but it's becoming more common."

I didn't really understand what that meant for me as a parent, though, until I went home, confused and frightened, with a week's worth of poorly assimilated training, a mountain of books, and an even bigger mountain of questions that tended to bubble to the surface at odd hours of the night. I scoured the books I'd been given, only to find that many of my questions weren't answered or were answered in general terms when I needed specifics. With the exception of one book, nearly all of the resources I looked at were written in the firm assumption that the child was old enough to communicate effectively about symptoms of highs or lows, and that the child could participate in his or her own care. Not true of my toddler! Eric was barely beginning to talk, and he certainly couldn't yet comprehend that the dizziness, headaches, shakes, and nausea meant something—and he wasn't even fully weaned yet, which complicated matters even further.

It didn't take long for me to realize two facts. First, there were very few resources out there for parents whose children were diagnosed as infants, toddlers, or preschoolers; and second, if this is the fastest-growing age group of children diagnosed with Type 1 diabetes, it would be helpful to have a book that would talk about the issues facing preschoolers as well as older children.

It also seemed to me that if I had trouble assimilating everything that was thrown at me in that week from hell at Maine Med—even after 15 years of working in medical publishing—parents who didn't have the same background I did would have just as much trouble or more. So, developing a book that reflected the parent's experience, as well as the doctor's knowledge, seemed like a good idea.

Another reason for developing this book is that treatment regimens for Type 1 diabetes are changing rapidly. The standard of care for Type 1 diabetes 10 years ago looks nothing like it does today, now that insulin pumps have become widespread, continuous glucose monitoring (CGM) is making inroads into the arena of diabetes treatment for children, and research and development efforts for a true artificial pancreas are at full steam. Some of the older texts I was given as references make no mention of insulin pumps, much less CGM.

At the time of this book's publication, Eric will have lived with diabetes for over 2½ years—well over half of his young life. At 4 years old, he is growing well, healthy, happy, curious, smart (and a little smart-alecky), and best of all, his diabetes is well-controlled by his insulin pump...at least till the next growth spurt! But it has been a rollercoaster ride—a learning experience of epic proportions that will continue for years to come until his father and I can gratefully, and probably with no small amount of anxiety, turn Eric's diabetes management over to Eric's keeping. While nothing will ever erase the memory of the October day that changed all our lives, I hope that other parents who pick up this book after going through a similar crisis with their teenager, child, toddler, or infant will take some measure of comfort in knowing that there's help available to teach you the ropes.

Elizabeth Platt
Buxton, ME
June 2011

PART ONE

The Basics

What is Type 1 diabetes?

Where does insulin come from,
and what does it do?

How does Type 1 diabetes develop
in a healthy pancreas?

More . . .

1. What is Type 1 diabetes?

Immune system

The collection of cells and actions that the body uses to fight off diseases, injuries, and toxic substances.

Pancreas

A gland of the digestive system that is responsible for releasing insulin, glucagon, digestive enzymes, and other hormones. The inability of the pancreas to produce insulin is the key problem in Type 1 diabetes.

Insulin

A hormone secreted by beta cells in the pancreas. Insulin is responsible for transporting glucose from the bloodstream into cells for energy.

Glucose

A simple sugar derived from carbohydrate foods that the body's cells use for energy.

The answer to this question is both very simple and a little complicated. We'll start with the simple: Type 1 diabetes is a disease in which the **immune system** attacks the cells in the **pancreas** that are responsible for producing **insulin**, the hormone that transports glucose into the cells. But unless you're already well versed in human biology or diabetes, that "simple" explanation probably isn't very clear, so we'll delve into it further. First, we'll describe what insulin does and why it's critical to our body's health and functioning; then, we'll describe our current understanding of what goes wrong to stop insulin production in the pancreas—the ultimate cause of Type 1 diabetes.

2. Where does insulin come from, and what does it do?

Whenever we eat anything, our digestive tract breaks the food down into smaller parts so that our intestines can extract the parts we need (glucose, proteins, fats, and various vitamins and minerals, among other things) and get rid of the parts we don't. One of the most important components of food is **glucose**, a simple sugar that the cells of the body depend on for instant energy. Glucose passes from the intestines into the bloodstream and circulates in the blood to the different tissues and organs throughout the body.

Here's where insulin comes into the picture. Insulin is a **hormone** secreted by cells in the pancreas known as **beta cells**. Insulin's job is to transport the glucose out of the blood and into the cells so they can make use of the energy it provides. There are a few exceptions to this rule (see the box), but for the most part, without insulin, the cells would starve, even if there were plenty of glucose in the blood just waiting to be used. A second role of insulin is to store any extra, unneeded glucose in the liver (where it is converted into a compound called **glycogen**) or in fat cells.

Because insulin is so crucial to providing energy to the cells, the beta cells in a healthy pancreas produce a little bit of insulin all the time so that cells in need of glucose are always able to get it—and when food is eaten, the beta cells release a flood of insulin so it can either transport the glucose to the cells, or store it in the liver and fat for later use if needed.

Sometimes, though, glucose from food isn't immediately available—either because we're asleep, or because we aren't able to (or don't wish to) eat food when we're awake. That's when the glycogen in the liver gets released, as a temporary stop-gap until we're able to eat food. If we're without food for an extended time (that is, longer than about 8 to 10 hours), the body reaches into its fat stores and starts burning those. This works for a short time, but the problem with burning fat instead of glucose for energy is that it releases a by-product called **ketone bodies** (**ketones** for short), which can be harmful in large amounts. We'll discuss ketones and the harm they do more later on (Questions 41–45), but for now it's enough to know that ketones are a sign of starvation—they're only present when the body is burning fat instead of glucose to get energy. And if there's still no food at this point, the body starts breaking down muscle as well.

Hormone

Chemicals released from gland cells that signal to other cells to perform certain functions or actions. Insulin, for example, signals to cells that they should allow glucose to pass through the cell membrane.

Beta cells

Cells within the pancreas that secrete insulin. In Type 1 diabetes, beta cells are attacked and destroyed by an autoimmune response.

Glycogen

Glucose that has been stored in the liver. Glycogen is converted back into glucose and released into the bloodstream if blood glucose levels fall too low.

Ketone bodies (ketones)

Acidic by-products of fat burning that can be harmful if generated for long periods of time.

Autoimmune disorder

A disorder in which the immune system mistakenly attacks the body's own cells as if they were pathogens.

Genetic predisposition

Having a gene or set of genes that makes one more likely to get a specific disease.

Trigger

An event that activates a genetic predisposition for autoimmunity, such as a viral infection or an exposure to toxic chemicals.

3. How does Type 1 diabetes develop in a healthy pancreas?

First and foremost, it's important to know that Type 1 diabetes most often results from an **autoimmune disorder**—that is, it's a disease in which the body's own defense system mistakenly attacks its own cells. It's also possible to get Type 1 diabetes if an injury or acute inflammation leads to failure of the pancreas, but far and away the most common cause of Type 1 diabetes is autoimmune destruction of pancreatic cells—so throughout this book, we're going to make the assumption that this is the source of your child's diabetes.

Autoimmune disorders like Type 1 diabetes generally occur in people who have a **genetic predisposition** for such diseases. But having this genetic predisposition doesn't automatically mean the person will develop a disease—it requires a **trigger** event, such as a viral infection or exposure to a chemical in the environment that arouses the immune system and gets it revved up so high that it begins to act against the body's own cells.

If we use the common analogy of immune cells as "soldiers" trying to protect the body from invasion, you can imagine that these "soldiers" have gotten an incorrect message that some portion of the body's own tissues are "invaders" that need to be destroyed, and they set about killing off any cells they find that match this description—never realizing that they're hurting their own "people." In the case of Type 1 diabetes, the victims of this "friendly fire" are the beta cells that make insulin.

In some children, the infection that triggers the autoimmune attack on the beta cells occurs a long time before the first signs of diabetes appear—it can show up many years after the fact, long after the triggering illness has been forgotten by the child and parents alike. In others, the transition from virus to full-blown diabetes is rapid, maybe even only a few weeks or months. We do not yet understand why the autoimmune response is so rapid in some children and so slow in others.

4. What happens once Type 1 diabetes develops?

In general, what happens is this: as less and less insulin becomes available because of the loss of beta cells, the child's **blood glucose** (the concentration of glucose circulating in the bloodstream) becomes abnormally high. The kidneys can't hold onto the excess glucose, so it begins to leak out into the urine. The urine takes on a sweet odor and becomes sticky when it dries. As the amount of excess glucose grows ever higher, more and more urine is needed to remove the overload, which leads to a cycle of excessive thirst and urination that is the symptom most often used to suggest the diagnosis of diabetes (see Question 6 for more on diagnosis). At the same time, none of this excess glucose is available to the cells because of the lack of insulin—the cells literally become starved for energy in the midst of the plentiful supply. So the body reacts just as it's supposed to when it's starving—by burning fat to provide energy (this is why weight loss is another common symptom of Type 1 diabetes). Burning fat, as we mentioned above, produces ketones as a by-product. Unless the diabetes is diagnosed and treated with insulin, the build-up of ketones leads eventually to **ketoacidosis** (see Question 44), which is a very serious, life-threatening condition.

Blood glucose (also blood sugar)

The concentration of glucose circulating in the bloodstream at any given time. Blood glucose is not constant but changes depending on the food you eat, the time of day, the amount of exercise you get, and other factors.

Ketoacidosis

A condition of low blood pH because of the presence of ketones in the blood. In people with diabetes, ketoacidosis generally occurs when a person has too little insulin for too long.

THE BASICS

Elizabeth's comment:

My son Eric was 18 months old when he was diagnosed with diabetes. He'd had a series of viruses in the months leading up to the diagnosis — one after another after another, a seemingly endless series of infections and fevers over the course of 3 months or so during the summer. The diabetes symptoms started in the fall about 2 months after this phase seemed to pass. We knew of one relative, Eric's paternal grandfather, who'd had diabetes, but we didn't know whether it was Type 1 or Type 2 — we'd always assumed it was Type 2, but he passed away years ago and we can't ask. Now, of course, we wonder whether Eric's grandfather may have had autoimmune diabetes.

Because of my work in health publishing, I knew that excessive thirst and urination were symptoms of diabetes. So when Eric started soaking through his diapers at night — and I mean FLOODING them — I started to become concerned. He was also asking for water a lot more. I checked it out on the internet and found that although thirst was clearly a symptom of diabetes, it could also be any number of other problems — or even just a passing phase! Eric didn't yet talk clearly enough for us to ask him how he felt, and his high level of crankiness could easily be put down to "terrible twos", so although I toyed with the idea of getting him checked, I didn't actually take steps to bring him to the doctor until his daycare provider said she was seeing the same thing during the day. When I heard that, I made an appointment with his pediatrician for the next day. I had my fingers crossed that he had a urinary tract infection or something else that could be cleared up with a round of medication, but I was sure in my heart of hearts that it was diabetes. I've never been so sorry in my life to be proven right.

But the real shock came when Dr. Foster told me to take him straight to the Maine Medical Center emergency department—Eric was in pretty serious trouble, and his symptoms and appearance didn't reflect the fact that he was in a true state of crisis. The pediatric endocrinologist on call (Dr. Olshan) met us at the door, ran the tests, and told me that Eric had a blood glucose of 569 and was in diabetic keto-acidosis, and that we'd be in the hospital for several days. I couldn't believe it. My son didn't even look sick—he seemed like a perfectly healthy toddler. Nothing I'd learned in my job prepared me for that.

5. What are the other types of diabetes? How are they different from what my child has?

There are a number of different forms of diabetes, and they're all similar in one respect: the primary symptoms are excessive thirst and excessive urination. But each disease is different in its causes and the problems occurring in the body.

Broadly speaking, there are two forms of diabetes: **diabetes mellitus** ("sugar" diabetes) and **diabetes insipidus** ("water" diabetes). Diabetes insipidus is a malfunction in the body's ability to concentrate urine rather than a disease of the pancreas—it bears no relation to Type 1 diabetes other than the name and the symptoms of thirst and urination. Type 1 diabetes is a form of diabetes mellitus, which is the general description of any form of diabetes in which the interaction of insulin and blood glucose has become impaired.

Diabetes mellitus itself is subdivided into several different types. Type 1, as we discussed in Question 1, is a complete failure of the insulin-producing cells in the pancreas, most often because of an autoimmune attack

Diabetes mellitus

Any form of diabetes in which the interaction of insulin and blood glucose has become impaired.

Diabetes insipidus

A form of diabetes related to the inability to concentrate urine. It is unrelated to diabetes mellitus.

Type 1 diabetes is a form of diabetes mellitus.

(this is why it's also known as *insulin-dependent diabetes mellitus* or IDDM—because a person with Type 1 diabetes is completely dependent on insulin to survive). **Type 2 diabetes** is the more common form of diabetes mellitus that has become widespread among American adults, and is showing up more often in adolescents as well (see Question 7). The two types have been traditionally regarded as completely different diseases, but recent research suggests they might be related—but we still don't understand how. So for the moment, it's useful to continue regarding them as separate situations.

Type 2 diabetes is a **metabolic disorder** in which the cells progressively lose their ability to respond to insulin (this is called **insulin resistance**). Most people with Type 2 diabetes still manufacture some insulin, but not enough to overcome their body's resistance to insulin's action—so in the end, a person with Type 2 diabetes still develops high blood glucose, just as in Type 1 diabetes. Although there's even a stronger genetic predisposition involved in Type 2 diabetes, it's a different set of genes affecting different biological processes, and there's no immediate trigger event. Instead, chronic, long-term exposure to being overweight (more on this in Question 23) combined with insufficient exercise gradually shifts a susceptible person into insulin resistance, then Type 2 diabetes. (Gestational diabetes, which occurs in pregnant women, is similar in nature but occurs for somewhat different reasons.) This is why some people with Type 2 diabetes, unlike Type 1, can manage their disease with a regimen of diet and exercise alone, or with oral medicines that reduce insulin resistance and lower blood sugar, without having to inject insulin.

There are also several lesser-known forms of diabetes mellitus. The first, commonly called "latent autoimmune

---

Type 2 diabetes

A common form of diabetes mellitus that occurs mostly in adults and is caused by the inability of cells to respond to insulin.

Metabolic disorder

A malfunction in the body's usual means of transporting and transforming food, water, and air into molecules that cells can use to live, function, and reproduce.

Insulin resistance

Loss of a cell's ability to respond to insulin appropriately.

diabetes in adults" or LADA, has unofficially been given the name "Type 1.5 diabetes" because it is very similar to Type 1—but it's a name not commonly used in the medical literature (although it's popular on patient-oriented web sites). Like Type 1, LADA is an autoimmune disease in which the beta cells are attacked by the immune system, but unlike Type 1, the disorder progresses very slowly—people with LADA often still produce enough insulin to meet their needs for years after diagnosis (this is one reason LADA is often initially misdiagnosed as Type 2). The second, called "maturity onset diabetes of the young" or MODY, is a monogenetic disorder that causes beta cells to fail to secrete insulin—not necessarily immediately, nor all at once. Having the gene for MODY doesn't mean that the individual with this gene loses all insulin, and some people with the gene are never diagnosed with diabetes at all. Many people with MODY who do get diagnosed do not show signs of diabetes until they're in their 50s, but most are misdiagnosed as having either Type 1 or Type 2. And the last is a combination of Type 1 and Type 2—that is, a person who is already unable to produce insulin on their own becomes insulin resistant, so that more injected insulin or oral agents are required to help keep their blood glucose levels stable. Many online and published resources erroneously call this insulin-resistant Type 1 diabetes "Type 3 diabetes" which, in the medical literature, is the name given to a completely different condition related to the brain's use of glucose; we're going to refer to it as "insulin-resistant Type 1 diabetes" in this book.

We'll talk a little more about insulin-resistant Type 1 diabetes in Question 60, but for the time being, unless your family has a history of Type 2 diabetes, it's probably not something you or your child need to worry about. All children become temporarily insulin resistant during adolescence because of the hormone shifts of puberty, but that will generally go away later on—and in any case, that's not what we're really talking about here. Pathologic insulin resistance, the type that's referred to as "prediabetes" in the general adult population, is something that develops over very long periods of time and usually can be prevented by eating a balanced diet and getting regular exercise. Just be aware that this is just one more reason why you'll need to pay attention to what your child eats now that diabetes is part of your life.

6. How is Type 1 diabetes diagnosed in children? What kind of doctor treats it?

Children may have different symptoms before diabetes is diagnosed, but the typical signs that point to diabetes are:

- Excessive thirst
- Excessive urination, particularly at night (that is, bedwetting in a child that hadn't previously been prone to it, or having to get up to pee in the night if that hadn't been occurring before)
- Tiredness, even when the child gets a full night's sleep
- Weight loss, even when the child is eating well
- Blurred vision
- Slow healing of cuts and bruises
- Irritability

What makes diabetes so hard to pinpoint right away is that these symptoms can all relate to other problems or can be part of ordinary growth.

Unfortunately, what makes diabetes so hard to pinpoint right away is that these symptoms can all relate to other problems, or can be part of ordinary growth. They're easy for parents to overlook or dismiss, particularly since the child might not think to mention them to the parent (and very young children are unable to express clearly that they're not feeling well). Symptoms may not all come at once, and they may come and go. So it's not at all uncommon for children with diabetes to be symptomatic for weeks, even months, before the pieces of the puzzle fall together and a diagnosis is made.

The initial diagnosis is almost always based on the results of either (or both) a urine test that looks for the presence of sugar and ketones in the urine and/or a simple blood glucose test looking for blood sugar of over 200 mg/dL. Either one of these results is good indication that the problem is diabetes.

Your child's diagnosis might have come from a visit to a pediatrician stemming from this collection of complaints, but your pediatrician is not going to be the doctor you work with for this particular disease. Diabetes is treated by an **endocrinologist**, a doctor specializing in hormonal disorders (insulin is considered one of the major hormones in the body). Children with diabetes are particularly challenging because their bodies are growing and their nutritional and metabolic needs are constantly changing, so most children diagnosed with diabetes will be referred to a **pediatric endocrinologist** if one is available.

7. How do my child's doctors know what kind of diabetes my child has?

Until fairly recently, diabetes in children has almost always been Type 1 diabetes, which is why it is often called "juvenile" diabetes. In very young children, ten years old or younger, it's still very unusual for a diagnosis of diabetes to be anything other than Type 1. So

It's not uncommon for children to be symptomatic for weeks, even months, before a diagnosis is made.

Endocrinologist

A doctor specializing in hormonal disorders.

Pediatric endocrinologist

A doctor specializing in hormonal disorders in children. Because children are growing, their hormones and metabolic needs differ from those of adults.

THE BASICS

your child *most likely* has Type 1 diabetes—and if there's anyone else in your family on either parent's side who has had Type 1 diabetes, it makes it that much more likely that Type 1 is what your child has.

However, many more children, primarily adolescents, are being diagnosed with Type 2 diabetes in recent years. If there's a history of Type 2 diabetes in your family and your child is school-aged, and especially if he or she is overweight, gets little exercise, and eats mostly foods that are high in sugar and carbohydrates (breads, potatoes, pasta, and other starchy foods), he or she could have Type 2 diabetes.

With most children, unless the child is overweight and has a family history of Type 2 diabetes, the diagnosis of Type 1 diabetes is generally correct. If there's any likelihood of Type 2, the diabetes team can use blood tests to check for the presence of **autoantibodies**. If they are present, it's nearly always Type 1; if not, usually it's Type 2. However, about 10% of children with Type 2 diabetes also show signs of autoantibodies, although they might not have *all* of the same autoantibodies that children who truly have Type 1 exhibit. And not all kids with Type 1 diabetes have identifiable autoantibodies. So the diagnosis of Type 1 versus Type 2 isn't necessarily cut and dried.

If you're unsure which type of diabetes your child has, it's important to speak to his or her diabetes team to clear up this confusion, because the two diseases are not managed the same way (see Question 5). Children with Type 1 diabetes *must* be given insulin, as their pancreas no longer makes insulin for them. Children with Type 2

Autoantibodies

Antibodies that trigger immune cell attacks against the body's own cells.

diabetes, however, may be treated with a program of dietary modifications, exercise, and if appropriate, medications that reduce insulin resistance and lower blood sugar, with a goal of avoiding the need for insulin injections. Neither form of diabetes can be cured, but Type 2 diabetes can be managed to avoid or decrease the need for insulin therapy in the long term.

8. What caused my child to get diabetes? Could I have prevented it?

Scientists do not yet know for certain what causes a child to get diabetes, but it's clear that there are a number of factors involved. One is genetics—a predisposition for diabetes often runs in families. There also seems to be a fairly strong environmental component. For example, in many instances, parents of children with Type 1 diabetes report that their child had a viral infection of some kind, often unusually severe, within a few months of the development of diabetes symptoms that led to the diagnosis. Some experts speculate that infection (possibly in combination with other environmental factors) triggers the autoimmune response in those with a genetic predisposition for it.

Ultimately the cause or causes of Type 1 diabetes are so complex, it's impossible to know whether any one factor could have been avoided or mitigated to prevent the child from developing the disease. Although some researchers are working on finding ways to halt the autoimmune response before diabetes is fully developed, for the most part there's nothing a parent can do once symptoms show up (and, of course, before the symptoms appear, you don't know there's a problem!).

Elizabeth's comment:

Of course I wondered, as all parents do, if I could have done anything differently to prevent Eric from getting diabetes. He was diagnosed just about the time I had started to wean him, so I thought, "Maybe if I'd kept nursing him, he'd have stayed healthy." And it was October, just about the time the sun gets too low in the sky here in Maine for people to make vitamin D, so after reading about the connection between diabetes and vitamin D deficiency, I wondered if he'd have stayed healthy if I'd been giving him supplemental vitamin D. In the end, I realized that I could drive myself bananas speculating and playing "what if", but it was all pointless, because for all I knew, none of those factors that I could have done something about had any relevance! Diabetes does run in Eric's father's family, and he had a series of infections, off again, on again, in the months before his diagnosis—and those were factors that I could do nothing about. I just had to finally accept that diabetes is just something that happened and I wasn't doing myself, or Eric, any good wondering why.

9. Is there any way to cure diabetes?

As of this writing, there is no cure for any of the different types of diabetes. This is not a reason to be discouraged or upset, however, because we have learned so much about these disorders in recent years that some scientists feel that it's only a matter of time before we find a definitive cure. We certainly have made tremendous advances in managing all forms of diabetes, whether it's through insulin regimens or dietary and exercise modifications. If you were to ask a person diagnosed with Type 1 diabetes as a child in the 1980s or even the 1990s, he or she would tell you that the management methods used today are very different from what was used 10 or 20 years ago. Research into all forms of diabetes is ongoing; some focuses on how to make current treatment methods easier and more effective (we'll talk about that more in the discussion of insulin pumps in Questions 37–39) while other research looks at ways to reverse the autoimmune response and restore the pancreatic beta cells to their original number and function. Many scientists and physicians feel hopeful that a cure is closer than ever.

10. What are the long-term effects of diabetes on my child's health?

One of the biggest concerns parents have when confronted with a diabetes diagnosis is the long-term impact of the disease. Many of them have heard of people losing limbs or eyesight to diabetes, and truly these are some of the more frightening results that come from diabetes that isn't well controlled. But here's the important point: *Diabetes can be controlled so that these health problems are less likely to occur.* It isn't always easy to achieve a steady state where blood glucose levels stay within the target range, and there will be high blood sugars as well as lows, but the important thing is that over time, the average blood sugar reading stays within a set range that your endocrinologist will help you determine.

Poorly controlled diabetes may certainly have some serious long-term consequences, including premature death (see Question 93 for the specifics). This is why maintaining good blood glucose control is so essential in a person with diabetes. But it's also important that parents understand that most of these problems result from many years of poor control. If your child has just been diagnosed, these complications are something you really don't need to worry about right now—in fact, worrying about them probably will only make your task harder. Certainly you need to be aware of them as the main reason why it's so important to work hard at developing good control—but if you can't "get it right" in the first few months, don't lie awake worrying about vision loss or heart disease, because they simply aren't likely to be an issue at this point in your diabetes journey with your child.

Later on, once you have an understanding of how to manage the disease day-to-day, you can start to focus more on how to prevent diabetes complications. It's important also that you learn enough about these complications—and teach your child about them too—so that you understand how serious they are, and how important prevention is, without being fearful or paralyzed by this knowledge. As we'll discuss in Question 70, sooner or later your child will need to take over diabetes management, and before that time comes, the child will need to thoroughly understand the consequences of poor control and to know that diabetes is a "non-negotiable" fact of life.

11. Will my child's diabetes get better or worse with age?

Type 1 diabetes doesn't change because of age—once the beta cells are gone, they're gone, and there's neither improvement nor deterioration to be looked forward to in the future. What *will* change over time is your child's insulin needs—those can fluctuate for many reasons, even something as simple as changes in the weather and temperature. If your child is suddenly having a series of high (or low) blood sugar readings and needs more (or less) insulin as a result, it's not a sign that he or she is getting "better" or "worse"—it's simply that today's insulin needs differ from yesterday's. One of the things that you as a parent—and your child too, eventually—will need to learn during the first few months, or even the first few years, post diagnosis is *how to recognize patterns of insulin use* so that you can predict (and hopefully avoid) the highs and lows.

We will talk more about the factors that can affect insulin requirements in the next section, **Managing Type 1 Diabetes in Children**.

12. Will my child develop normally and live a normal life?

A child whose diabetes is managed well absolutely *will* develop normally and live a normal life. The best way that you as a parent can make sure that this happens for your son or daughter is to do three things:

First, learn all you can about diabetes and how to manage it, and make sure your child is a partner in his or her diabetes management as early as possible. You might be surprised at how young you can start—children who are old enough to read numbers can begin to learn how to read their blood glucose levels, and even toddlers learn that when they feel a certain way, they need to ask for juice.

Second, educate not only yourself, but all those who will be supervising your child at school, daycare, camp, and so forth about what diabetes is, what the warning signs of low blood sugar might be, and what to do if an emergency arises. Ideally, you'd have support from daycare providers and school officials, but this isn't always the case, so be prepared to advocate for your child.

Third, connect with a diabetes support network. There are a number of them listed in the Appendix, and any of them can offer you valuable information and support when you need it (and you *will* need it!). Raising a child with diabetes can be a tremendous challenge, but help is available. And there's help out there for your child, too—especially if your child is school-age or older, and likely to have tremendously conflicted feelings about the diagnosis.

We also recommend that you do not refer to, or think of, your child as "a diabetic," and try to discourage others in your family (as well as teachers, caregivers, friends, etc.) from using that term as well. One of the biggest issues children with diabetes face is the label "diabetic"—it makes them feel like they're defective, incapable, or less than what they should be. Your child's physical health depends, to a certain extent, on his or her ability to accept that diabetes is a condition that certainly needs considerable attention, but doesn't define how he or she lives life (see Question 67).

Diabetes needs considerable attention, but it doesn't define how your child lives life.

13. What makes diabetes different for children than for adults?

We could write an entire book answering this question alone, but for the time being we'll mention just a few specific factors that make the experience of having diabetes different for children than for adults.

Growing. At the risk of stating the obvious, children grow; adults do not. The energy needs of a body that is still developing are different from those of an adult. For one thing, insulin needs can fluctuate wildly from month to month, week to week, or even sometimes day to day, particularly when a child is going through a growth spurt. Human growth hormone, the hormone that promotes growth spurts, causes cells to become temporarily insulin resistant, which can contribute to trends of high blood sugars in growing children.

Eating habits. Anyone who has ever tried to coax a young child to eat vegetables knows that children do not eat food based on whether it's good for them or even because of the flavor—they choose based on familiarity, appearance, scent, and (unfortunately) how often they see it on television or in their friends' lunchboxes. Children have to be trained in making healthy food decisions, and it can be a pretty tough road for parents—particularly parents who themselves have difficulty making healthy choices (we know just as well as anyone that just because we *can* make these choices, doesn't always mean we *do*!). Moreover, where most adults have established a pattern of three meals a day with small snacks in between, children often eat erratically—sometimes grazing throughout the day, other times turning down food altogether for no obvious reason. This kind of patternless eating can have an effect on blood sugar readings and insulin needs. Older kids may also sneak food or deliberately eat high carbohydrate foods out of rebellion.

Maturity. A sign of emotional maturity is the ability to look at a planned course of action, forecast whether it will have good or bad results, and decide whether the consequences are something you're willing to live with *before* you act. Unfortunately, this capability is something we have to learn through trial and error—through the experience of *not* doing it and living through the consequences. Children learn it only when adults teach it to them, often repeatedly—if you've ever told your child, "You can only have a video if you first clean up your room," over and over (only to have the child complain when the video is denied because the room wasn't cleaned), you know exactly the lesson we're talking about.

An adult with diabetes usually "gets it" that failing to take care of diabetes will lead to very unpleasant health problems and a shorter life; a young child with diabetes is incapable of fully grasping that message—it simply doesn't compute. Older children and teenagers may understand it in the abstract, but they often have trouble relating the idea to their own situation until they reach full emotional maturity—and when they do, they frequently rebel against the knowledge or reject the reality of their circumstances (see Question 99).

Fewer habits to break. It may seem like the deck is stacked in favor of adults, and to a certain extent it is—but children do tend to have one advantage over adults when it comes to dealing with diabetes. Unlike adults, children don't have decades' worth of habits, patterns, routines, and accumulated health issues weighing them down when they're learning to handle their diabetes. An adult who has spent the past 35 years drinking soda for breakfast is going to have to consciously make the effort to break that habit as part of diabetes management—but most children, particularly pre-teens, have their routines and choices set by their parents, who are likely to make healthier decisions for their children than they might make for themselves. In very young children, it's possible to prevent the formation of problem habits before they even start—and young children, especially, lack the emotional issue of comparing life before diabetes to life post-diagnosis, simply because they don't remember a time when diabetes wasn't a part of life.

Overall attitude. Another place children generally benefit by their youth is attitude. Unlike adults, children tend to "live in the moment" a lot more and be less burdened by worry — they don't play doomsday scenarios in their heads. While this can be a drawback as well as a blessing (because part of regulating diabetes is figuring out how your blood sugar should respond in 2 hours to the things you're doing or eating right now, which is hard to do when you're focused on the immediate), children are much more likely to be accepting of their situation — the younger the child, the greater the acceptance. The changes that accompany a diabetes diagnosis might lead to depression, anger, denial, and grief in a teen or an adult, but similar emotions are considerably less likely — or less profound — in a child. Parents should realize, though, that their own emotions about the diagnosis may influence their child's response; we'll talk about this more in Question 90.

Elizabeth's comment:

As difficult as it is caring for a toddler with diabetes, I'm thankful Eric was diagnosed so young. He'll never know a routine that doesn't include regular blood glucose monitoring and insulin. The sense I've gotten from people I've talked to is that the older you are when you're diagnosed, the harder it is to adjust because you're simply more set in your ways, and you're more inclined to resent the unfairness of it all. The emotional burden is harder for older kids, and that makes it harder for the parents too. I've been told that most teens with diabetes go through a rebellion phase where they ignore their insulin needs and blood sugars. I hope I'm not being naïve in imagining that it will be far less difficult for a kid like Eric, who will have spent his whole life living with diabetes, than for a child who is still trying to adjust to diabetes while going through adolescence. I guess I'll find out when we get there.

PART TWO

Managing Type 1 Diabetes in Children

How is Type 1 diabetes managed?
Will my child need insulin shots?

Can my child's diabetes be controlled
with diet and exercise instead of insulin?
Should I be worried about my child's weight?

What is a "diabetes kit"? What does it contain, and
why does my child need one?

More . . .

14. How is Type 1 diabetes managed? Will my child need insulin shots?

Since there is currently no cure for Type 1 diabetes, the only treatment available is to replace the insulin that is no longer being produced in the pancreas. And it must be given by injection rather than pills because insulin is destroyed by the acids and enzymes in the stomach. So, yes, your child will need either insulin "shots" (also called **multiple daily injections** or **MDI**) or an insulin pump (see Question 37). However, there's a lot more to it than just injecting a specific amount of insulin now and then, and many different factors are involved in determining the correct dose at any given time, so we usually speak of "managing" diabetes rather than "treating" it.

The goal of diabetes management is to mimic the action of the pancreas by providing a **basal** supply of insulin—that is, a certain low, continuous, but variable level of insulin that is present in the blood 24 hours a day—along with a **bolus** of insulin given at mealtimes that "floods" the system with insulin in response to food, just as a healthy pancreas would. We'll talk more about basal and bolus insulin in Question 29.

What makes this tricky for the parent or the child with diabetes trying to achieve this goal is that, unlike a healthy pancreas, a person doesn't have the hormonal signals telling him or her how much insulin to put in to take care of the glucose in the blood. The only information you have about how much insulin your child needs is the snapshot provided by using a **blood glucose meter**, and there are limits to what that snapshot can tell you. In essence, diabetes management requires children with diabetes (or their parents, at least until the children are old enough to do it themselves) to make an educated guess as to how

Multiple daily injections (MDI)

The treatment protocol in which insulin is manually delivered using syringes.

Basal insulin

The low level of insulin that is always present in the bloodstream.

Bolus insulin

A dose of insulin given all at once in response to food intake or to correct a high blood sugar.

Blood glucose meter

A mechanical device that uses a drop of blood to assess current blood glucose levels.

Management of Type 1 diabetes is not an exact science but is more about pattern recognition.

much insulin is needed based on what the child's blood sugar is currently, what the patterns of blood sugars have been recently, and the carbohydrate content of food that he or she has eaten (or is about to eat). Management of Type 1 diabetes, in short, is not an exact science—it's more about pattern recognition. Even more complicated is the need to adjust the insulin dose based on the level of physical activity expected for hours *after* the insulin dose.

What parents of children with diabetes need to learn (and to teach their children eventually) is how to make those educated guesses accurately enough that they maintain blood sugars that are neither too high (leading to long-term complications) nor too low (leading to short-term crisis or even coma).

A child with Type 1 diabetes always needs insulin to be injected into the bloodstream through the skin in one form or another—there's no getting around it. In the past, that always meant regular, repeated injections of insulin with a syringe or insulin pen—and for many families that's still the best option. However, there are new technologies available that are helping some children to avoid that regimen. **Insulin pumps**, which deliver a predetermined dose of insulin at regular intervals and allow for additional doses to be programmed in response to meals and elevated blood sugars, are one such technology that is becoming more broadly available to even very young children. Right now, an insulin pump combined with **continuous glucose monitoring** (a device that keeps a real-time assessment of blood glucose levels and sounds an alarm when they fall outside a pre-set range) is about as close to an **artificial pancreas** as one can get—although medical device companies are continually refining this combination in the hopes of developing a true artificial pancreas.

Insulin pump

A mechanical device that gives basal and bolus doses of insulin as programmed by the pump user via a cannula inserted under the skin.

Continuous glucose monitor (CGM)

A mechanical device that monitors blood glucose levels and issues a warning when levels fall below or climb above the ideal range.

Artificial pancreas

A mechanical device, still in development, that combines insulin pump, CGM technology, and other features to function much like a real pancreas.

Insulin pumps have both advantages and disadvantages that we'll talk about in depth in Question 38.

When it comes to treatment, the part that you may be most concerned about is just how active you as a parent are going to have to be. Most parents are perfectly comfortable when their child's pediatrician gives them a liquid medication at a set dose that the child takes two or three times a day for a week to treat an ear infection, but when it comes to diabetes management, the level of involvement is considerably more intense. It's very unnerving to be told you'll need to continually monitor every bite the child eats and calculate the dose of medication yourself, particularly considering the number of variables that can affect how much insulin is really needed (see Question 33). But here are some things to keep in mind when you feel overwhelmed:

- Over time, your child will learn to take care of his or her own needs—you will not always have to be the principal caregiver. When the transition occurs depends on how young your child was at diagnosis, but sooner or later it *must* happen for your child to become an independent, functioning adult.

- Caring for your child's diabetes will very quickly become a matter of routine if you look at it as a set of new habits you need to acquire.

- Many other parents have been through this exact same situation, and quite a few of them were less prepared than you are to handle it—so if they can do it, you can too.

- You have a team of people ready and able to help you develop the skills you need, and there are many resources and agencies you can turn to for support (we list some of these in the Appendix).

Elizabeth's comment:

The idea of giving your kid shots four or five times a day can be frightening to a parent—I know it was for me, especially since I've had a long-standing phobia of needles. And the computations that are needed to calculate how much insulin to give can seem confusing at first. But if you set your mind to the idea that you will learn this new skill because you have to—and you DO have to, because your kid's life literally depends on it—you'll get it down pretty quickly. Keep in mind that your child's diabetes team members know that this is new and frightening, and they will be there to help you through the first scary weeks. And I can't emphasize enough that there are plenty of organizations and support groups out there to help. Use them! I got incredible support from the Juvenile Diabetes Research Foundation and TuDiabetes.org in the weeks after Eric's diagnosis, and it made a world of difference. I learned an amazing number of tips and tricks in the first year of dealing with Type 1 diabetes, and I'm sure there are plenty more to come.

15. Can my child's diabetes be controlled with diet and exercise instead of insulin? Should I be worried about my child's weight?

Type 1 diabetes is always controlled with insulin. A child with Type 1 diabetes is able to eat any foods offered as long as adequate insulin is given to process the carbohydrates in that food.

Type 1 diabetes is always controlled with insulin.

Even so, it's beneficial to the child to strive for a diet that minimizes sugar and other simple carbohydrates and emphasizes healthy foods—vegetables, fruit, lean meats, and so on—over junk food. Easier said than done, even without diabetes in the mix—we know! But considering the long-term danger of insulin resistance, which can greatly complicate Type 1 diabetes later on (see Question 60), the sooner you can promote healthy eating for your child, the better. This may mean you have to rethink your entire family's food choices, which we know can be difficult—but many parents use a diabetes diagnosis as an opportunity to promote a healthier diet for the whole family.

And while regular exercise is good for any child, in Type 1 diabetes it's especially important, again because healthy exercise habits can limit the possibility of insulin resistance in the future and help maintain a healthier cardiovascular system so that long-term complications are less likely. But there are considerations of how exercise impacts insulin usage that must be accounted for; we discuss these in Question 68.

Because there is so much information (and misinformation) in the popular media about Type 2 diabetes and its relationship to obesity, many parents think they need to keep their child's weight "in control"—but that's actually not the case! In Type 1 diabetes, the child's weight is not a contributing factor to the disease. Your goal as a parent is to try to keep your child at a weight that is healthy and in keeping with his or her body type, age, and developmental phase. We caution parents—particularly parents of girls, for reasons we'll discuss in Questions 44 and 99—not to obsess about the child's weight but focus more on keeping good blood glucose control, making sure the child eats healthy foods, and encouraging regular exercise. If those conditions are met, and if there is no strong family history of being overweight, chances are that your child will weigh exactly what he or she is supposed to—and, more important, will be healthy.

16. What is a "diabetes kit"? What does it contain, and why does my child need one?

Children with Type 1 diabetes are susceptible to extreme highs and lows in their blood sugar (see Questions 17 and 18), because their bodies are no longer able to respond appropriately to changes in blood glucose. As a result, the child will always need to carry certain tools so that such extremes can be treated at any time, day or night, when the child is not at home. These tools can be collected into an insulated bag or backpack to form the child's diabetes kit.

At bare minimum, the kit should include:

- a blood glucose meter, used to determine current blood glucose, and test strips for this meter
- alcohol wipes for cleaning the finger prior to testing
- a finger-stick device to draw blood for testing
- rapid-acting insulin, so that insulin can be injected should the child eat or have high blood sugar for other reasons
- a mechanism for injecting insulin, such as a syringe — and keep in mind that the kit should contain at least one syringe even if the child uses an insulin pump, so that insulin can be delivered in the event of a pump failure
- fast-acting simple carbohydrates to address low blood sugar, usually in the form of glucose tablets, juice boxes, candy, or similar sugary foods
- a notebook or logbook to record blood sugars, insulin doses, carbohydrate consumption, and any unusual factors such as illness or hot weather, to help establish patterns of insulin use

- a glucagon kit for rapid treatment of severe hypoglycemia (see Question 48)
- urine ketone strips, or a blood ketone meter and strips, for testing ketone levels (see Questions 41–45)
- a card containing the child's emergency contact information and diabetes alert information
- a set of sick day guidelines, as supplied by your diabetes center
- a pen

Optional, but very useful, items to add to the kit include a calculator; a carbohydrate counter such as the Calorie King book; Band-aids, Q-tips, antiseptic ointment, and cotton balls for caring for pricked fingers; spare syringes or finger-stick needles; spare insulin pump supplies; favorite toys or books to distract a young child who doesn't want to receive a finger-stick or injection; snack foods, such as crackers or granola bars, to tide the child over if a meal is delayed or missed on a busy day.

This list may seem endless, but most of the items on it are small and fit easily within an ordinary backpack or even a medium-sized diaper bag. A diabetes kit enables your child and you to have the tools you need to prevent or treat extreme high or extreme low blood sugars. Without it, your child is unable to eat, play, or sleep outside the home in safety, because changes in blood glucose levels can occur unpredictably and without warning, and if you don't have the tools at hand to treat these changes, your child could have a health crisis.

Elizabeth's comment:
The Juvenile Diabetes Research Foundation offers newly diagnosed children with diabetes a free "Bag of Hope" that is tailored toward children of different ages. We found that the

backpack they sent was the ideal container for Eric's diabetes kit, not only because it includes a special, insulated pocket for insulin vials, but also because it has the Foundation's name on it, and that lets people know what the backpack is for. We've had odd looks from people when they see us reaching into a backpack and pulling out a vial and syringe, but they see the JDRF logo and it saves us a lot of complicated explanations.

17. What is hypoglycemia, and why should I be concerned about it?

"Hypoglycemia" means "low blood sugar" (hypo = low, glycemia = blood sugar). Simply put, a person with **hypoglycemia** has insufficient glucose in his or her bloodstream for the cells to get enough energy. Hypoglycemia is especially worrisome when it comes to brain function, as the brain above all cannot function without a certain amount of glucose in the bloodstream, and it will shut down if it becomes starved for glucose. Severe hypoglycemia, unless it's quickly corrected, can lead to seizures, coma, and (if untreated) brain damage or death. While it's unlikely that your child is going to face any of these consequences, as a parent of a child with diabetes, you need to learn how to recognize the signs of hypoglycemia and how to treat it so you can prevent these concerns.

Hypoglycemia
Low blood glucose levels.

Simply put, a person with hypoglycemia has insufficient glucose in his or her bloodstream for the cells to get enough energy.

With a low blood sugar, one generally feels dizzy, fatigued or weak, craves sugar, and sometimes gets cranky or irritable. If your child is an older school-age or adolescent child (say, 8 or older), it's likely that he or she will quickly learn to recognize hypoglycemia and can tell you that he or she is "low" so you can take action (assuming the child isn't able to do something about it on his or her own). In younger children, though, parents absolutely must watch for signs of hypoglycemia and coach the child about what to say when they feel a certain way. Especially in children who aren't talking comprehensibly (those under the age of 3 or 4, particularly), it's crucial to learn your child's nonverbal cues. If you're lucky, you'll have a child who "acts out" by having tantrums or tears when he or she is low—it's a great deal easier to recognize hypoglycemia in such children than in those who become quiet and inattentive as their blood sugar drops.

If you see your child acting oddly or staring into space, check his or her blood sugar.

Be aware that even if your child is old enough and verbal enough to recognize and ask for help with hypoglycemia, it doesn't always mean that he or she will always do so. Children, particularly adolescents, sometimes dislike bringing attention on themselves with regard to health matters, so they might hesitate to speak up even when they know there's a problem (especially when they're in school; see Questions 76 and 78). Moreover, low blood sugar can sometimes affect not only the child's judgment about what to do, but their ability to take action even when they know they need help! Even adults with diabetes find that lows can sneak up on them if their attention is captured by something else for a long period of time, and once blood sugar becomes too low, it's very easy to become too fatigued or disoriented to treat it yourself. *If you see your child acting oddly or staring into space, check his or her blood sugar,* even if this is normally something you trust the child to do without prompting.

Elizabeth's comment:

In the first months after Eric's diagnosis, we were very fortunate that he responded to low blood sugar with extreme crankiness—he'd frequently wake from a sound sleep screaming if he dropped below 60. This cost me a lot of sleep, since anytime he cried in the night I assumed he was low and run to get the meter, which fairly often showed that he wasn't low at all—many times, the problem was teething, not hypoglycemia! More recently, though, he's had some lows that he didn't wake for—on at least three occasions in the past 6 months or so, it was just sheer chance (or maybe mother's instinct?) that I found him low while he was sleeping. I've been told by my diabetes educator that people with diabetes can become insensitive to lows if they experience a number of them in a short time span, and this was probably what happened. So if he's had a few lows, I tend to pay more attention to his blood sugar when he's asleep as a result. You learn pretty quickly what is normal for your child when sleeping, and what's not—sweating profusely, cool, clammy skin, shallow breathing, those are the things that trigger me to reach for the meter when Eric is sleeping.

18. What is hyperglycemia? Why might my child have a high blood glucose reading?

Hyperglycemia is the condition of having too much glucose in the bloodstream (hyper = high, glycemia = blood sugar). "Highs" can occur for a number of reasons, but the most common reason is that too little insulin has been given to the child to counterbalance the amount of carbohydrate he or she has taken in. The obvious remedy is to give more insulin. But parents should be careful not to immediately inject insulin when they get high readings without making sure that it's not a "false high".

Here are some reasons you might get a high reading . In some cases, high readings might occur even when your child actually has the right amount of insulin on board:

Dirty hands. Food residue on the child's finger can sometimes fool the meter into delivering a higher reading than is actually the case. You should make a habit of washing your child's hands—or at very least cleaning

> **Hyperglycemia**
> High blood glucose levels.

the test finger with an alcohol wipe—before pricking the finger for a test. Don't be shy about testing again, or testing a toe instead of a finger, if you get an unexpected high reading.

Too little time has passed for the insulin to have fully affected blood glucose levels. So-called "rapid acting" insulin begins to work on blood glucose within 15 minutes after injection, but it still takes a certain amount of time for it to complete its work—so if your child eats too soon after having the insulin (or if the child eats before the insulin is given), the blood sugar will become higher because food is being absorbed at faster rate than the insulin is able to act on it. The ideal situation is to give a bolus of insulin about 10–20 minutes before the child starts eating, but that works best in school-age children who are old enough to reliably eat everything they're given. For preschoolers and toddlers, who may eat less than a full meal or refuse to eat altogether, it's safer to give the bolus just before, during, or even after the meal to make sure they eat all of the carbs you expect them to eat. A blood sugar reading taken within 2 hours or so of a meal eaten immediately after (or before) insulin administration can be relatively high without posing any real danger to the child's health and well-being. This is why most pediatric endocrinologists will advise parents not to test at all within a 2-hour time span of a meal and insulin injection (unless there are symptoms of hypoglycemia), and to give additional insulin only if it's needed to cover any carbohydrate intake for any food eaten within that time frame. The concern is that if you correct a high blood sugar reading when there's already insulin in the bloodstream from a previous correction or a bolus given less than 2 hours beforehand, you'll end up overcorrecting and causing a low when the glucose from the meal has been used up.

Insulin that has lost its effectiveness. Once you open a bottle of insulin, it's good for about 28 days—and that time is shortened if it is regularly exposed to temperatures above 80° F. If you're using diluted insulin for a toddler or infant, its shelf life is even shorter—2 weeks at most. So it's important that you pay attention to the lifespan of the insulin you're currently using.

If you use syringes and your child suddenly starts getting high readings every time you check, ask yourself the following questions:

- Are you drawing from a vial or using a pen that's been open more than 4 weeks?
- Are you unsure how long your current vial or pen has been open?
- Has the vial or pen you're using been out of the refrigerator and exposed to warm temperatures (>80° F) for an extended period of time (more than a few hours)?

If you answer "yes" to one or more of these questions, it's possible that the insulin is no longer viable. In this case, you should discard the current vial or insulin pen and open another one, making sure to mark the expiration date on the new vial or pen with a marker.

Pump failure. Insulin pump users have a separate set of possibilities when it comes to figuring out why blood sugar is running high (see Question 37). Hyperglycemia in a pump user may occur for several reasons:

Air bubbles in the pump tubing. A few, tiny bubbles here and there won't likely cause hyperglycemia, but larger bubbles, or clusters of many small bubbles, could cause a problem. Bubbles mean that air, not insulin, is being delivered, so the pump must be disconnected and primed to remove the bubbles. It's also a good idea to check your child for ketones if you spot multiple small bubble clusters or large air bubbles in the infusion set tubing. Be aware that bubbles often occur because the insulin is too cold when you put it into the reservoir; when filling a pump reservoir, it's important that insulin be at room temperature.

A compromised insertion site. Pump cannulas made of plastic can crimp, bend, or become blocked, especially if they've been in place for more than 2 days. If the cannula gets fully blocked, the pump is supposed to sound an alert identifying the lack of insulin flow, but if it's incompletely blocked, the alert may not sound — yet the child still isn't getting enough insulin. The short-term solution is to change the insertion site (and check for ketones), but if you find this problem happens repeatedly, you might wish to talk with your pump manufacturer about other types of insertion sites that could work better.

Inadequate basal rate and/or carb ratio settings. Children's needs for insulin change as they grow. If you find that you're having repeated problems with high blood sugars but see no evidence of either bubbles or pump site problems, it could simply be that it's time to re-evaluate the child's pump settings — particularly if the high readings are consistently only slightly out of the target range and respond well to corrections given via the pump.

Medications. A number of medications can raise blood sugar, sometimes substantially; a list of such medications is available at www.diabetesincontrol.com. Some of these medications are commonly used in children, particularly those that relieve cold symptoms, bronchitis, asthma, or allergic reactions (prednisone, albuterol, and epinephrine, to name a few). See Question 65 for more on medications that affect blood sugar.

Adrenaline. Most parents know that excitement or fear causes the release of adrenaline, a stress hormone that raises heart and respiratory rate—you have only to watch a child opening birthday presents to know that! What many parents may not realize is that it also produces high blood sugar as a (usually temporary) side effect. If your child is highly excited, nervous, or agitated, you may see high blood glucose readings. We've even seen this in children who are involved in sports, where you'd think their blood sugar would be low, not high—the excitement and adrenaline of going onto the soccer field can offset the need for additional energy needed for running and kicking. The effect, however, lasts only a short while.

19. Why is it important to test my child's blood sugar regularly?

In a healthy adult or child, it's normal to have a blood sugar level of about 80 when we wake up in the morning—and usually, right after we've eaten a meal, it goes up to around 150–180, depend-

> **HELPFUL TIP**
> When you take your child's blood sugar, prick the side of the finger rather than the fingertip. It hurts less!

ing on what's eaten. A healthy person's blood sugar stays within that range because we have systems in place to make sure it doesn't fall too low or soar too high—but in a child with Type 1 diabetes, those controls are no longer available, so it's up to the child's parents (or the child if he or she is old enough) to keep blood glucose levels within the healthy range. The only way a parent can know the need to correct blood glucose levels that are too high or too low is to check them regularly.

Depending on your child's age, your diabetes team will give you a **target range** that sets the limits of how low and how high your child's blood sugar should go. The

Target range

The range of blood sugar levels that are considered acceptable for a child with diabetes.

ranges are less aggressive in younger children, whose brains are still developing rapidly and may be more sensitive to damage by low blood sugar, and more aggressive in older children, whose brains are more developed and who are also more capable of detecting the onset of low blood sugars. The range of acceptable blood sugars also may differ at night versus during the day. So, for example, your child may have a range of 100–200 daytime and up to 250 at night as a toddler, 80–180 daytime/220 night time in preschool, and perhaps 70–140/200 as an adolescent.

Hypoglycemia can come on very quickly, and severe hypoglycemia is very dangerous.

Hypoglycemia can come on very quickly, and severe hypoglycemia is very dangerous, so it's important that you take steps to prevent low blood sugars. The best way of doing this is to develop a consistent routine around monitoring blood glucose so that you can learn your child's metabolic patterns and how to compensate for them—preventing lows that occur at the same time every day might be as simple as making sure your child sits down with a small snack at that time. Likewise, if your child is regularly showing high blood glucose numbers at a certain time of day, it may mean his or her insulin regimen needs to be adjusted—but unless you check and record the blood sugar numbers *routinely* at approximately the same intervals every day, you will not be able to see this pattern. High blood sugar readings are not quite as immediate a concern as low ones (unless they're *very* high and accompanied by ketones—see Question 41), but over time, continuous high blood glucose can be very damaging to your child's health (see Question 93). Monitoring routinely and adjusting for high readings is the best way to limit the likelihood of long-term health problems.

Elizabeth's comment:
We've always tested regularly, always before meals and bedtime, and at times more often. I do a moderate amount of "gut check"

testing when he's napping or at night, and several times it's helped me to quickly treat some rather scary lows. There was one time when Eric was deeply asleep, and I noticed that he was sweating a lot—not normal for him, and a sign of a potential low. Usually he wakes up when he's low but not always, and he'd been pretty tired that day, so I got out the kit and tested him. Good thing, too, because he was at 38! I grabbed a juice box and woke him enough to drink it, and got most of it into him before he started having a small seizure. At that point I switched to fudge syrup, which he was less likely to choke on, and within about 30 seconds the twitching stopped. I kept feeding him syrup and eventually got him back up to his normal range. We figured out later that we'd given him too much insulin to cover some ice cream he'd had at the county fair earlier in the day.

20. How often should I test my child's blood sugar during the day? How often at night?

Generally, it's best to test your child as soon as he or she gets up in the morning, then again before each meal or snack, and finally once more at bedtime for a total of five to seven times per day. It's usually not necessary to test overnight unless your child's blood glucose patterns haven't been fully determined yet;

> **HELPFUL TIP**
>
> For nighttime testing, instead of turning on the lights (and potentially waking your sleeping child) or trying to juggle a flashlight, get a headlamp similar to the ones used by miners and cave explorers from an outdoors supplier like L.L. Bean or REI.

parents of newly diagnosed children usually are advised to test once or twice during the night, then gradually ease off from nighttime testing as they learn their child's nighttime blood glucose patterns. (We suggest, however, that parents do a midnight and 3 AM check at least once a month even after the child's patterns are established — if only because patterns change!) There are some situations that call for more frequent testing, such as:

- A newly diagnosed child who is in or just beginning the "honeymoon phase" (see Question 35)
- A child who is sick with a fever, particularly if he or she is vomiting (see Question 63)
- A child who has an unexpectedly low reading generally warrants re-testing within 15 minutes to confirm the number is within the target range after treating with carbohydrate
- A child who has an unexpectedly high reading generally warrants re-testing a couple of hours later to make sure that the treatment for a high blood sugar worked well
- A child who is participating in sports or strenuous exercise, particularly in warm temperatures (above 80° F)
- A child whose behavior changes in ways that could indicate a high or low blood sugar (see Question 25 for a list of signs and symptoms to watch for).

As with anything, there are pros and cons you should be aware of when it comes to testing. On the "pro" side, regular testing is an important part of maintaining good control of your child's diabetes, and good control, in turn, will help your child avoid health complications later in life (as well as preventing extreme blood sugars that can be an immediate concern). Regular testing can help you to head off an emergency situation, such as an unexpected low. But on the "con" side, focusing on testing *too* much can keep parents in a constant state of worry and anxiety, which gets transmitted to the child—who may, as a result, come to fear or resent having a finger stick. Testing repeatedly at night also means a lot of unnecessary lost sleep for you and your child, unless you're fortunate enough to have a very sound sleeper. What's more, individual blood glucose tests don't give more than a snapshot of blood sugars at any given time, unless you put them together to look for patterns (see Question 21).

When it comes to testing, we encourage parents to test at least five times a day, at the times we mentioned earlier; test at least once during the night until you're comfortable that your child's blood glucose is stable overnight; test more frequently if your child is sick or in a physically or mentally stressful situation (such as playing in a soccer game or taking an important test at school); and to "follow your gut" and test if you see your child acting oddly. Most important of all is to try to maintain a sense of the routine while you're doing it—finger sticks are simply part of living with diabetes, and the more you accept this and act like it's perfectly normal, the more your child will, too.

Elizabeth's comment:

We made an extra effort to act as if finger sticks were no big deal—even stuck ourselves so that Eric could see it was a normal, ordinary thing. Within 3 months of his diagnosis, all I had to do was say, "I need a finger" and he would hold out his hand for a finger stick without a second thought. Within 6 months, he had even done his own finger stick a few times—once with no prompting from me, as a way of letting me know he wanted his breakfast! All this when he wasn't quite 2 years old. It was pretty amazing. We do try not to be too compulsive about it—in the first few weeks after his diagnosis, and again when he started the pump, we were testing an awful lot, but once things settled down, I'd say we were testing about seven or eight times a day. He didn't get quite to that same point of being casual about injections, though. Sometimes he'd hide from me and act like he was playing hide-and-go-seek, but it was clear he was trying to avoid being "poked." I let him pull the syringe plunger out of the used syringe to make a popping noise as a reward after the poke, and that's something he seemed to enjoy. Now that he's on the pump, he really dislikes the occasional injections he gets when the pump doesn't work right, so playing "pop goes the plunger" is that much more necessary. I'm not sure it's going to work for him much longer, though!

21. Is it possible to test too much?

Yes. Anxiety can turn parents into compulsive testers, and that's not good for either you *or* your child. No matter how worrisome the highs and lows of diabetes may be, if you find yourself reaching for the meter every hour or two, day and night, you're testing too much. Such frequent testing may be a sign either that you need to work with your diabetes educator to obtain more consistency in blood glucose levels, or that you need to talk to a counselor to lessen your anxiety levels (particularly if you're testing repeatedly despite getting readings in the target range). Your child's life—and yours!—should not revolve around diabetes that much.

Working with your diabetes team to achieve greater control may be one answer if the numbers are truly so widely variable that you need to test that often to avoid highs and lows, but if anxiety rather than fluctuating blood glucose is what's driving you to use the meter repeatedly, then counseling from a therapist familiar with the issues facing parents of children with diabetes may be another answer.

Another clue that you're over-testing is if you find yourself getting charged for the extra test strips you buy because you've exceeded the coverage your insurance company offers. While insurance companies can be stingy with test strips (some will only authorize four tests daily, which is clearly not enough!), even the most comprehensive insurance coverage will likely support at most 10 tests a day (that is, ~300 strips per month). If you test more than that, your insurer may refuse to cover additional test strip purchases for that month without a notice from your endocrinologist stating that the testing is needed because of problems controlling blood sugar levels.

22. What is an "A1c test", and what does it tell me about my child's diabetes?

The **hemoglobin A1c test**, also called the "A1c" or "HbA1c" for short, is a blood test that measures the amount of **glycohemoglobin** in the blood. Glycohemoglobin is a protein that forms in the blood when glucose binds to **hemoglobin** (the blood protein that carries oxygen in the bloodstream) in the blood. In people without diabetes, glycohemoglobin makes up about 5–6% of the total hemoglobin in the blood. However, the more glucose there is available, the more glycohemoglobin will form, so you would expect a person with diabetes who has higher than normal glucose levels in the bloodstream to similarly have higher than normal glycohemoglobin present.

What makes the A1c test useful is that when hemoglobin forms in red blood cells, it remains in circulation for 60 to 90 days. That means that the amount of glycohemoglobin in a sample of red blood cells is representative of the average amount of glucose in the blood over the previous 2 to 3 months. So, by looking at the percentage of glycohemoglobin in that sample, your diabetes team can get a pretty good idea of how well your child's blood sugars have stayed within the target range during the past 3 months. In short, it's a "big picture" measure of whether the treatment regimen is working well.

For a person with diabetes, an A1c of 7% or lower is considered ideal, as this measurement corresponds to an average blood glucose level of about 150 mg/dL. A reading of 8 is considered fair, as it represents an average blood glucose of about 180. Anything above that, however, is an indication that blood glucose levels are generally too high, and will probably lead to some changes in the treatment regimen. (Our own practice considers any

Hemoglobin A1c test

A blood test measuring the amount of glycosylated hemoglobin in the blood; the test gives a good indication of how well blood glucose is controlled over a 3-month time span.

Glycohemoglobin

Hemoglobin to which glucose is bound; a measure of long-term control of diabetes mellitus. Also called **glycosylated hemoglobin**.

Hemoglobin

A protein in blood that carries oxygen to the cells.

reading above 7.6 to signal a need for changes, depending on the child's age.)

There are some drawbacks to the A1c test. First of all, it doesn't change quickly when the treatment regimen is altered — it's an *average*, so it takes a fairly significant amount of time before the value starts to change. So if your child was diagnosed with an A1c of 9% or above, and a month later still has an A1c of 9%, don't be discouraged — remember that this reading reflects weeks, possibly even months, of excessively high blood sugars related to the slow decline in insulin production. It may take several months of insulin treatment before the A1c value goes down to your desired target.

Second, many parents treat the A1c reading as a test of their capability in managing their child's diabetes, and feel as though they've "let down the team" when an A1c value comes back higher than expected. But the test is not done to assess parents' skill at managing diabetes; it's done to review whether blood glucose has been stabilized so that the treatment regimen can be reassessed if necessary. More often than not, a high A1c is a sign that the insulin regimen is insufficient, usually because the child has grown since the last time it was calculated. In very young children (under age 5) who are given insulin injections after or during a meal rather than before because they aren't reliable about eating, it's not unusual for A1c readings to fluctuate or remain consistently above 8%. Young children also have less aggressive target range, so their higher blood sugars lead to higher A1c readings. As the child gets older, you'll be able to forecast what he or she will eat more accurately and give insulin before the meal, not after — and that will help keep blood sugar from climbing too high, so that the A1c value goes down.

23. What are carbohydrates, and why are they important in diabetes?

In Question 2, we talked about how glucose is the fuel that cells need to function properly. **Carbohydrates** are compounds in food that are the major source of glucose. In ordinary terms, they are sugars and starches in food, and when broken down in the stomach and intestines, they supply glucose.

Carbohydrates

Compounds in food that are broken down into glucose.

But carbohydrates aren't all created equal: some are simple—think potatoes, juice, soda, and anything made with white flour or sugar—and some are complex (whole grains, vegetables, and raw fruit fall in this category). The difference between the two forms lies in how fast the food breaks down from its original form into glucose. Simple carbs tend to break down more quickly; complex carbs take more time. As a result, simple carbs make blood sugar rise rapidly, while complex carbs make blood sugar rise more slowly (this is what's referred to as the glycemic index, covered in Question 53).

Carbohydrates are important to diabetes because the amount of insulin needed by a person with diabetes at mealtimes depends largely on how much carbohydrate that person consumes in the meal. As a parent, you will need to learn how to calculate the amount of carbohydrate in your child's food so you can use it to determine the bolus insulin dose (see Questions 29 and 31). You also need to know the difference between simple and complex carbs so you can make effective choices should your child become hypoglycemic, and so that you can better judge the time frame for bolus insulin doses given before meals (see Question 33).

24. What do I do when my child's blood sugar is low or high?

In a healthy person, symptoms of mild hypoglycemia are resolved simply by eating any kind of food (although a carbohydrate is usually what people reach for because it breaks down into glucose quickly). Once the glucose gets into the blood stream, the brain has the energy it needs and the symptoms go away.

In a person with diabetes, however, it's not so simple. The symptoms might truly mean that there's too little sugar in the blood, but it could also be a sign that there's plenty of sugar but the body is releasing stress hormones for another, unrelated reason (a geometry test later in the day). These hormones create many of the same symptoms as appear from hypoglycemia. This is why a child with diabetes who is experiencing symptoms of dizziness, shakiness, nausea, and rapid heart rate needs to use a glucose meter to determine whether blood sugar is low or high, so they or their parents can choose the correct treatment.

Treating hypoglycemia

In the case of hypoglycemia (usually a reading below 100 in infants or toddlers, 80 in school-age children, or 70 in teens), the correct treatment is to have your child consume something with a simple carbohydrate in it. The rule of thumb for treating a low is "15 carbs, 15 minutes" (e.g., you give your child 15 grams of fast-acting carbohydrate and test again in 15 minutes after consumption to make sure that the blood sugar reading has risen). Juice, candy, or chocolate syrup generally works best with children, so parents are advised to keep some handy at all times. And we mean it when we say *at all times*—your child's diabetes kit, your medicine chest, and your car should all contain some form of fast-absorbing carbohydrate (a juice box or glucose tablets), and juice, hard candy, small tubes of cake gel, or glucose tablets should go wherever your child does and be within easy reach should the child become "low". Hypoglycemia needs to be treated *immediately*, and you can't treat it if you don't have some sort of fast-acting carbohydrate handy. With younger children, we increase our safety zone by treating blood sugars that are 70 to 100 as well, because we're concerned that they might not be as adept as recognizing the symptoms of low blood sugar.

It may seem counterintuitive to reach for sugary foods if you've conditioned yourself to believe that children with diabetes should be *avoiding* sugar, but it makes sense when you realize that your child's tissues and brain are starved for glucose. The brain, remember, doesn't need insulin to take up glucose, so the sooner you get your child to eat some sugar, the faster he or she will feel better. Juice, cake gel, syrup, and candy are recommended because the simple sugars in these foods don't need to be broken down much to pass into the bloodstream—in fact, some of it will pass directly into the bloodstream through the mucous membranes of the mouth, without needing to go through the digestive tract. This is especially handy for small children who become cranky and uncooperative when low—you can rub frosting on the gums or squirt juice in between the teeth and lips to get fast results.

Crash

Sudden development of hypoglycemic symptoms related to a rapid drop in blood glucose to hypoglycemic values.

Hypoglycemia can sometimes come on very quickly, causing what's often called a "**crash**"—that is, a sudden, unexpected appearance of hypoglycemic symptoms. If this happens (particularly if you've recently administered insulin), you may need to take emergency action. See Question 46 for more details on hypoglycemic emergencies.

Hypoglycemia can sometimes come on very quickly and lead to a "crash."

Elizabeth's comment:

I don't know about other parents, but my two favorite treatments for lows are juice boxes — the small ones with the little straws that poke through the foil into the box or pouch — and Hershey's chocolate syrup. The little juice boxes with the straws are ideal because they have the right amount of carbs in them — most have 13–16 carbs, which is close to the 10–15 carbs that's usually recommended — they don't need refrigeration, so they can be stored just about anywhere, and if my son gets combative and refuses to drink the juice, I can squeeze the box and squirt it into his mouth through the straw. That's especially useful if he presses his lips together! As for the Hershey's syrup, that's good for lows because I've never met any child who wouldn't eat it if offered, and a table-spoon provides enough carbs to stop any episode of low blood sugar in its tracks. Except when he's super cranky, Eric will always take syrup — that's not always the case with juice. The books I've read also recommend Skittles, but because he's just a toddler, I'm afraid he might choke, so I don't use hard candy — although it would probably work if he were older.

Treating hyperglycemia

When blood sugar is high, it's important to take a look at the big picture and determine *why* it might be high before you treat. As we noted in Question 18, a high reading doesn't necessarily mean you must give your child insulin. Sometimes the reading is exaggerated by food residue on the skin; other times the reading is high because insulin you've already injected hasn't had time to work yet or is ineffective; and sometimes they're high from sheer excitement. But if you can rule out these pos-sibilities and confirm that your child is legitimately high, the next step is to determine how much insulin your child currently has in his or her system, and from there calculate how much insulin you need to inject so that you can bring your child's blood glucose reading down to the normal range. The amounts will vary from child to child depending on age, weight, and metabolic needs, so you'll refer to the instructions given to you by your diabetes educator in determining the amount to give.

When blood sugar is *very* high, that is, 240 mg/dL or higher, it's important to check for ketones before you go ahead and treat. The level of ketones present can indicate a need for greater amounts of insulin. High ketones are considered an emergency (see Question 43), and ketones in pump users may be a sign that the pump isn't functioning correctly, so be prepared to consult with your diabetes care provider as well as your pump manufacturer if you find ketones above the level your provider tells you is acceptable but are unable to find any obvious reason for the stoppage of insulin flow (more on this in Question 38).

25. What signs or symptoms should I be watching for?

When your child's blood glucose level is too low or too high, your child will experience physical symptoms that indicate there's an imbalance of insulin to blood glucose. Although these symptoms vary somewhat from person to person, in general, you can expect to see some or all of the following:

Low blood sugar
- Irritability, confusion, and anxiety
- Trembling, weakness, palpitations, and sweating
- Hunger, sugar cravings
- Headache

With extreme low blood sugar, seizures and coma are possible.

High blood sugar
- Excessive thirst and urination
- Warm, dry skin
- Fatigue, tiredness, and dizziness
- Headache, blurred vision

In severe hyperglycemia, the following symptoms might also be seen (and they should be considered an emergency, as they often signal the onset of diabetic ketoacidosis—see Questions 44 and 45):
- Abdominal pain
- Difficulty breathing
- Vomiting
- Rapid heart rate with weak pulse
- Loss of consciousness

These symptoms might sound frightening, but the fact is, most parents know their child's "normal" behavior well enough to spot changes before they become severe, particularly once they know what they're looking for. If your child acts oddly, becomes unusually irritable or quiet, or complains that he or she doesn't feel well, it's worth testing to see if there's a problem with blood glucose levels.

Elizabeth's comment:

Eric is normally a sunny, high-energy child. It's pretty easy to know when he's low, because he gets lethargic and grouchy, and he sweats buckets. When he's sleeping, his breathing becomes very shallow, his skin becomes cool and damp, and he gets pale if he's low. Highs are a little harder to detect because unless he's high for a while—several hours at least—he doesn't show it. This was one reason we didn't catch his diabetes sooner, I think, because the symptoms he did show were also typical "terrible twos" sorts of signs, and were pretty easy to explain as teething or 2-year-old tantrums. But I've started to realize that when he's high, he goes way beyond "high-energy"—he's practically manic. If he's high at bedtime, he can't settle down—flops all over the bed like a fish out of water, and that's a clue that I need to test him. And he asks for water a lot and soaks his pull-ups—that's another clear sign that he needs insulin.

26. When do I need to call the endocrinologist or diabetes clinic?

Different clinics offer different guidelines for when parents should reach out for assistance, but in general, it is a good idea to get in touch with your endocrinologist or clinic staff under the following circumstances:

- If your child is vomiting and unable to keep down juice (this may be a medical emergency if the child has a low blood sugar prior to vomiting—see Question 63);

- If your child has ketones greater than 0.6 mmol/L (for a child on an insulin pump, ketones greater than 0.3 mmol/L);

- If you have had a series of unexplained lows or highs (>240) and are unsure how to adjust your insulin regimen to accommodate these variations.

- Keep in mind that although doctors and nurses usually have on-call staff, "off hours" calls (weekdays before 9 AM or after 5 PM, or weekends) are reserved for issues that are time sensitive and can't wait until normal hours.

27. What is meant by "tight control"? Is that something we need to try for?

"Tight control" means maintaining blood glucose levels within a very limited range so that the A1c readings stay at around 7% for extended periods of time. The value of tight control is that people with diabetes who are able to keep themselves in this range experience fewer long-term health problems. In children, tight control is difficult, if not impossible, to achieve because of all the variables affecting their blood sugars. Nevertheless, it's a good idea for parents to have the goal of developing tight control in their child to help him or her develop good habits.

Here are some important recommendations:

Regular meals will make your life a lot easier. Children with diabetes, as much or even more than all children, benefit from healthy lifestyle and eating habits. Growing children should eat regularly. With young children, that usually means breakfast in the morning, followed by a small mid-morning snack, then lunch at mid-day, with another snack in the afternoon and dinner in the evening — and for some children, a glass of milk or peanut butter and crackers before bedtime is also important to keep their blood sugar elevated overnight. The problem arises with "grazing," which is common in young children and teens. In this situation, a parent must make decisions about insulin doses without having complete information. That is, if the child eats within 2 hours of a previous meal, you do not know how much of the previous meal has been absorbed, nor do you know how much insulin remains from the previous injection. To avoid this problem, it is best to eat no more frequently than every three hours. Bear in mind that a balance of carbohydrates, fats, and proteins are essential to stable blood sugars as well — a diet high in carbohydrates, particularly simple carbohydrates, doesn't lend itself to good control of blood sugar (we talk more about this in the section **Feeding a Child with Diabetes**).

Get into the habit of reviewing the blood sugar and insulin doses to look for patterns. Your child's insulin therapy is individualized—no two kids will need the same amount of insulin administered in the same way, and even your own child's needs will change over time. The only way to determine how much insulin is required at any given time is to know your son's or daughter's metabolic patterns—and to figure those out, you'll need to know how their blood sugar levels respond to their day-to-day activities and their food intake. Most people use a log book of some kind to write down blood sugar levels, carb intake, and insulin dosage, and we encourage parents to do this—but remember also that your blood glucose meter has a memory function, so if you forget to write down a reading, you can go back and look at the history to jog your memory. The same goes for insulin pumps—boluses, pump priming, and the date you last changed the reservoir are all kept in the pump's memory for several days.

Keep an eye on the ratio of basal insulin to bolus insulin. Basal insulin (see Question 29) usually makes up at least 40% of the total insulin dose your child receives each day, and generally no more than 50% in most children (although, as with most factors in diabetes treatment, individuals vary). So, for example, if the total amount of insulin your child receives each day is 15 units, about 6 to 7 units, but probably no more than 7.5, should be basal insulin and the rest (~9 units) bolus insulin. If the child receives less than 40% or more than 50% from the basal dose, blood sugar readings are likely to be much less stable, which could put the child at risk of serious complications.

Don't go overboard! Some parents become obsessive about maintaining tight control in their children. While their hearts might be in the right place, taking a hard-line approach to the disease is rarely productive—usually the opposite, in fact, as the child quickly tires of hearing parents continually fretting about blood sugar readings, carb counts, and so forth—and sooner or later rebels against the effort to maintain tight control, whether openly or covertly. And since part of being a parent of a child with diabetes is teaching the child healthy techniques for managing the disease, alienating your child through too great a focus on tight control ultimately undermines your ability to help him or her in the long run.

As much as you may try to keep your child within the healthy blood glucose range, unexplained highs and lows happen to all people with Type 1 diabetes from time to time—adults as well as children. It is simply not humanly possible to imitate the action of a healthy pancreas perfectly, and parents will experience nothing but heartbreak and frustration if that's what they try to do. So our advice is, do the best you can, understand that your best won't be perfect, and focus on being a loving parent while striving for the best blood glucose control you can obtain.

INSULIN

28. How do I administer the insulin used to help control my child's diabetes?

Because your child is no longer able to produce insulin in the pancreas, you will need to administer synthetic insulin on a regular basis to meet the child's insulin needs. This is done by one of several possible methods: periodic **subcutaneous** injections using a syringe or insulin

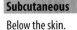

Subcutaneous

Below the skin.

pen, or subcutaneous infusions with an insulin pump. We'll talk more about pumps in Question 37, but for right now, when we talk about insulin administration, in general we're talking about syringe delivery. Older children and teenagers can often use insulin pens, but the amount of insulin delivered by a pen does not allow for the fine adjustments that are generally required in very young children.

A few things to know about insulin and how to administer it:

- Once opened, insulin can be kept at room temperature (59° to 80° F) for up to 28 days without spoiling. Room temperature insulin is often more comfortable to inject, so it's perfectly acceptable to keep it in a cabinet if the overall ambient temperature isn't too high. However, temperatures higher than 80° F will gradually cause the insulin to lose effectiveness, so you should make sure to keep your insulin in the refrigerator in climates or seasons where room temperature is above 80° F.

- Even if it's not opened, insulin will spoil if kept too long at room temperature, so unopened insulin vials should be stored in the refrigerator. If you are purchasing insulin by mail order, be sure to check that the cold packs are still cold when it arrives so you can be certain it hasn't spoiled. Insulin should **never** be frozen, however, because once thawed, it will clump and become unusable.

- You can still use insulin that has been at room temperature after 28 days in a pinch, but it may not be as effective as a fresh vial, so it's not recommended. Ideally, parents should make a point of always keeping an unopened vial of insulin in the fridge to replace an open one just in case something unexpected happens, like a heat wave or a power outage. If you get stuck without a fresh vial after your current vial expires—the pharmacy is closed for the night or on a holiday—you can use the expired insulin, but monitor your child's blood sugar carefully and replace the vial as soon as possible.

- If your child is very young or physically small and you are delivering insulin with a syringe, you may need to dilute the insulin with sterile saline in order to be able to deliver small quantities. The smallest syringe available delivers a minimum of 0.5 units of insulin, but small children may need as little as 0.1, so diluting the insulin makes it easier to deliver these tiny doses by syringe. Your healthcare provider will give you instructions on how to dilute insulin, but you should be aware that diluted insulin has a much shorter shelf-life than full-strength insulin. Mix up a new vial and discard the old vial of diluted insulin after two weeks of use, or if your child is experiencing unexplained, repeated high blood sugars near the end of the mixture's life expectancy (>10 days).

- Generally, one should **not** use the same syringe to administer long-acting and short- or rapid-acting insulins. Mixing the two causes the action time of the long-acting insulin to change, so you will be unable to predict when the basal dose is no longer in effect. However, you can give separate injections of long-acting and short-acting insulin (at different sites) at the same time (see Question 30 for more on different forms of insulin).

- If you're using an insulin pump, you will be administering *only* short-acting insulin to your child in the pump. However, you will need to keep some long-acting insulin on hand in the refrigerator as a backup in case of a pump failure.

- Insulin needs to be administered under the skin into fat, not into a blood vessel or a muscle. Both blood vessels and muscles should be avoided when giving an injection because injecting insulin into vessels and muscles hurts more, and it also makes insulin absorb more rapidly, potentially leading to lows and highs.

- The best locations for injecting insulin are the places in the body that have the most subcutaneous fat: the abdomen, thighs, buttocks, and the fleshy part of the upper arms. The abdomen is a good location, but it can be uncomfortable or even frightening for very young children, for whom the thighs or buttocks are generally better sites. As children get older and start to do the injections themselves, they'll likely find the abdomen to be more convenient and less painful, and switch to this location on their own.

- Avoid injecting the same location repeatedly, as this can cause the fatty tissue to develop lumps that some people find uncomfortable or unsightly. It's usually a good idea to alternate sides of the body each time you inject your child to avoid coming too close to a prior injection site.

29. What is meant by "basal" and "bolus" doses of insulin?

A healthy pancreas delivers insulin in two ways: first, it emits a small amount of insulin continually to keep blood glucose in balance—if it did not do this, blood sugar would gradually rise because the liver releases glycogen to provide energy for the brain while we're asleep. Second, when a meal is eaten, the pancreas rapidly increases the amount of insulin it secretes to keep pace with the glucose entering the bloodstream from the digestive tract, then tapers off once blood glucose drops to normal levels.

In people without diabetes who aren't insulin resistant, blood glucose generally doesn't fall below 65 mg/dL or rise above 150 mg/dL.

Diabetes treatment seeks to imitate the action of a pancreas as much as possible. For this reason, your child will be given both a **basal** dose of insulin that acts all day, just as the pancreas emits small amounts continually, and a **bolus** dose of insulin that counteracts the carbohydrates consumed in meals and snacks.

Basal insulin doses for children are generally very, very small—as little as one-fifth of a unit per hour, or even less for infants and toddlers. Such doses clearly can't be given by syringe, even if a parent were tireless and dedicated enough to want to deliver them hour after hour—the child simply couldn't tolerate that many injections! So if you're using syringes, you'll be giving your child two different forms of insulin: one long-acting (for the basal dose) and one short- or rapid-acting (for the bolus doses). We'll talk more about these different forms of insulin in Question 30.

Bolus doses of insulin are administered when the child eats any food containing carbohydrates, or when the child's blood sugar is high and needs correction. The size of the dose is calculated in relation to how much carbohydrate was eaten (see Question 31), or (for a correction bolus) how high the blood glucose level is in relation to the maximum level in the child's range. While a healthy pancreas can tailor the amount of insulin to the child's precise needs, a parent can't do the same, so a bolus dose of insulin must be calculated according to the best information a parent has about what the child needs (see Question 33).

30. What kind of insulin will my child be using?

As mentioned in Question 28, if your child is getting insulin via syringe, there will be two forms of insulin administered. The basal insulin is usually provided in the form of **long-acting insulin** (for example, Lantus® or Levemir®). There are a number of different forms of long-acting insulin, and each form has a slightly different **activity profile**—that is, the timing of when it starts to act in the body and when it reaches peak activity—but all of them have a roughly 12- to 24-hour-long duration in the body. Most forms start working within about an hour of injection.

Basal insulin is also sometimes supplied with a form of insulin called **intermediate-acting insulin** (NPH), which (as its name implies) only lasts for a portion of the 24-hour day, usually 12 to 16 hours. These forms of insulin must either be injected twice per day to provide a basal dose for 24 hours, or be used only overnight, which is sometimes useful for children who find it too uncomfortable to wear an insulin pump during the night.

Bolus insulin is generally supplied by using a **rapid-acting insulin** (Novolog®, Humalog®, or Apidra®), which starts working within 15 minutes, lasts roughly 4 hours, and peaks from about 1½ to 3 hours. Rapid-acting insulins are particularly useful in very young children whose food intake is unpredictable because its speed of action enables parents to inject the insulin after the child finishes eating without fear that blood sugar will climb excessively high before the insulin starts to work. But if your child's eating habits are more predictable, your child might instead be prescribed a **short-acting insulin** (also called regular insulin) which has a slightly

Long-acting insulin

Insulin that has been synthesized to have a 24-hour activity profile.

Activity profile

The timing of a form of insulin's activity levels, including its peak activity and duration.

Intermediate-acting insulin

Insulin that has been synthesized to have an 8- to 12-hour activity profile.

Rapid-acting insulin

Insulin that begins to act within 15 minutes and generally lasts about 4 hours, peaking within 2–3 hours.

Short-acting insulin

Insulin that begins to work within an hour and lasts about 4 hours.

longer duration but which starts to work much more slowly, requiring as much as 30 to 45 minutes in the body before it starts lowering blood glucose.

The type and brand of insulin your child is prescribed will depend on many factors, including whether you're using a syringe or a pump (and whether the pump is used 24 hours or less than that); how old your child is; whether the child is willing or able to follow instructions about meals, snacks, and insulin delivery schedules; and, to a certain extent, the personal preferences of your endocrinologist and the coverage offered by your insurance.

31. What is meant by "carb ratios"? How are carb ratios determined?

Meal bolus doses of insulin are given based on the amount of carbohydrates a child eats, but the amount of insulin per gram of carbohydrate differs from child to child, and even from meal to meal in the same child. **Carb ratios** (more correctly "insulin-to-carb ratios") are the measurement of how many carbohydrates can be processed by 1 unit of insulin at any particular time of day.

Carb ratios

The amount of insulin used for each gram of carbohydrate eaten.

Because the body's hormones and metabolism changes during the course of the day, children generally need more insulin to process carbohydrates in the morning, when hormonal influences are strongest, than they do at noontime or in the evening. So the carb ratios at breakfast will likely differ from the ratios used for lunch and dinner.

To give you an example, the carb ratios for Elizabeth's son Eric when he was diagnosed at 18 months old (when his insulin was delivered via syringe) were as follows:

1 unit of insulin per 25 grams of carbohydrate at breakfast
1 unit of insulin per 35 grams of carbohydrate at lunch
1 unit of insulin per 35 grams of carbohydrate at dinner

Given that a child of 18 months only rarely eats as much as 35 carbs ("carbs" = grams of carbohydrate) in a sitting (10 to 20 carbs is more common), this meant that his parents were often giving him less than a full unit of insulin for a meal—sometimes as little as 0.3 or 0.2 units. Because such miniscule amounts can't be measured in a syringe, the insulin had to be diluted with saline to 10% strength, allowing the quantity delivered to return to whole numbers again (so that a dose of 1.0 unit contained 0.9 saline and 0.1 insulin). However, as children grow, the amount of insulin needed to process the same number of carbohydrate becomes steadily (and rapidly) greater. At age 3 years and 6 months, Eric's carb ratios looked more like this:

1 unit of insulin per 19 grams of carbohydrate at breakfast
1 unit of insulin per 23 grams of carbohydrate at lunch
1 unit of insulin per 28 grams of carbohydrate at dinner

A child at 3 eats a lot more food than a child at 18 months (30 or 40 carbs in a meal isn't unusual for him at this age), so even if he weren't on a pump, Eric's parents could measure the insulin in a syringe and be more-or-less accurate. But as you can see, the amount of insulin in relation to his carb intake has gone up too—where he used to have to eat 25 grams to get a full unit of insulin, now he only has to eat 19. Added height and weight means he has millions more cells needing insulin to transfer glucose into them. When you consider this fact, it makes sense that his carb-to-insulin ratio should change over time.

Carb ratios are determined by starting with a general knowledge of how much insulin a child of a particular age and weight might use in the course of a day. As we mentioned in Question 29, about 40% of the total insulin dose in a day is basal insulin, which means that the remaining 60% is used for processing the glucose from food we eat. The average amount of insulin used by children of particular ages has been known for quite some time, so a general set of carb ratios can be determined by your endocrinologist based on that knowledge. These ratios are a starting point, and you and your child will likely go through weeks or months of "tweaking" by your diabetes team before you settle on ratios that will keep your child in a good range. And as we showed above, these ratios will change over time as your child grows and requires more insulin to process the same amount of carbohydrate.

It's worth noting that upon starting pump therapy when he was 28 months old, Eric's ratios increased a bit—that is, his insulin requirement went *down*, not up. Because the pump is able to deliver doses as small as 0.05 units and is much more precise in measuring the dose than even a careful parent can be, diluted insulin wasn't needed, so the change in ratios represented an improvement in his control. The fact that his basal insulin was delivered continuously in small amounts throughout the day, and could be tweaked to give more or less basal insulin as his activity levels called for it, instead of in a single long-acting dose also helped to improve his control.

32. What is the "correction factor," and how is that determined?

At times, your child's blood sugar will be higher than it's supposed to be, and you'll need to correct it by giving your child an extra bolus of insulin. But how much insulin should you give the child? You want to give enough to bring the blood sugar level back into the target range, but not so much that the blood sugar will go too low.

The **correction factor** is a ratio of insulin to blood glucose so that for every X mg/dL of glucose over the upper limit of your child's range, he or she would receive 1 unit of insulin. It's important to know that for many children, a slightly less aggressive correction factor is used at night, when parents might be concerned that overcorrection could bring the child low while asleep.

Correction factor
The amount of insulin needed to correct a specific proportion of blood glucose above the upper limit of the acceptable range.

To use Eric as an example again, at the time this book was first written (January 2010), his correction factor was 1 unit per 180 mg/dL of blood glucose. Since his parents were certainly not about to let him get 180 mg/dL above his range, the factor was divided by 10 so that they could dose him with 0.1 units for every 18 mg/dL above his upper limit, which was set at 180. Thus, if Eric's blood sugar was between 181 and 199 mg/dL, he'd get 0.1 units of insulin to correct; from 200 to 218, he'd get 0.2; from 219 to 236, 0.3; and so forth. The series of correction doses in relation to specific ranges of high blood sugar measurements is referred to as a **correction scale**.

Correction scale
The series of correction doses in relation to specific ranges of high blood sugar measurements.

Correction factors, like all other numbers in Type 1 diabetes, are subject to change as your child grows. Over time, your diabetes team will alter the child's correction factor to suit these changing needs. Again, Eric's example is useful here: by mid-2010, his correction factor had been lowered to 1 unit of insulin per 140 mg/dL, a change of 40 mg/dL in less than 6 months. By year's end, it was set at 120 mg/dL.

33. How do I calculate how much insulin to give my child?

As we mentioned earlier, determining a dose of insulin can be confusing for the parent at first, because so many factors influence the child's needs at any given time. But there is a certain "method to the madness" that we can describe in general terms.

Calculating basal insulin doses

Dose determination for basal insulin is fairly straight-forward. Based on your child's age and weight, your endocrinologist will start the child on a dose of long-acting insulin (if using a syringe) that is appropriate and will monitor how the child's blood glucose levels change during the night for a week or so, adjusting the dose if the nighttime readings are too high or too low. If your child is on a pump, the process is similar—a nighttime basal rate will be calculated based on what it's expected your child will need, and this rate will be programmed into the pump. Depending on how the child responds, the programmed rates will be adjusted up or down on a trial-and-error basis until you and your team are secure that enough insulin is being delivered to keep the child in range without developing hypoglycemia.

Your child's diabetes crisis and its aftermath are covered by the Family Medical Leave Act.

In both cases, you and your diabetes team will periodically review the overnight and morning numbers to see if growing, honeymoon (see Question 35), or other factors alter that dose. And in both cases, you probably will need to get up two or three times in the night to check blood sugar, so if you can arrange your work schedule to allow for time off or a shorter work day during this period, you'll be much better off. Speak to your child's endocrinologist about having a conversation with your employer if you are concerned this could be a problem at work, and remember that your child's diabetes crisis and its aftermath are covered by the Family Medical Leave Act (see the Appendix). But after a while, you will find the dose that works best for most circumstances, and you will be able to suspend the multiple night time checks after a few weeks.

Bear in mind that when your child gets sick, starts or finishes a honeymoon period, or has a growth spurt, the dose that was working fine may suddenly be too much or too little—unexpected lows or highs in the morning (or in the night) will be your first clue that something has changed. When you first begin managing your child's diabetes at home, don't be afraid to consult your diabetes team about temporarily raising or lowering the dose until the illness, honeymoon, or growth spurt passes; after a while, you'll become comfortable making those decisions without their input.

Calculating bolus insulin doses

Unfortunately, when it comes to calculating bolus doses of short-acting insulin, there is no hard-and-fast rule regarding how much insulin a child gets. Giving insulin isn't like giving an over-the-counter medication where the manufacturer prints a dose for a child of a certain age or weight—although those parameters do help provide general guidance. Every person metabolizes food and uses insulin differently, and insulin needs change depending on time of day, activity levels, the weather, the child's overall health (aside from the diabetes), how much sleep the child has had—even the child's mood and energy levels have an impact. Giving insulin is more of an art than a science, and as a parent you'll find that it's mostly a matter of making educated guesstimates informed in part by a rough knowledge of your child's general pattern of insulin use.

If this sounds worrisome, remember that your diabetes team will be helping you to learn the ropes. Over time, you will learn how to calculate appropriate doses. But understand that while you're learning your child's patterns of insulin use, it's *essential* that you keep good records of what your child eats, when your child eats, how much insulin you gave for each meal, and above all, the pre-meal blood glucose levels. These pieces of data are what will help you determine your child's patterns as well as calculate insulin doses. Many people with Type 1 diabetes use log books or log sheets similar to the one shown here to keep track of daily insulin and carb intake, and to note any lows or highs.

When it comes to calculating a bolus dose, there are certain variables you need to assess prior to giving the dose:

1. The very first thing to consider is the child's current blood sugar. Before you even consider giving a bolus dose, you *must* test blood glucose levels. If you give a bolus without testing first, and your child's blood sugar is already in range or low, you could trigger hypoglycemia. Understand that blood sugar can sometimes change very quickly, so if you tested an hour ago and are only now getting to the point of delivering the bolus, test again to be certain the child's blood sugar hasn't dropped in the meantime. On the other hand, if you don't test and the child's blood sugar is higher than the acceptable range, the dose you calculate will be

Date	12:__	1:__	2:__	3:__	4:__	5:__	6:__	7:__	8:__	9:__	10:__	11:__	12:__	1:__	2:__	3:__	4:__	5:__	6:__	7:__	8:__	9:__	10:__	11:__
						AM												PM						
Blood Sugar																								
Grams of Carb																								
Insulin for Carb																								
Insulin to Correct																								
Total Dose																								
Lantus Dose																								
Ketones																								
Date	12:__	1:__	2:__	3:__	4:__	5:__	6:__	7:__	8:__	9:__	10:__	11:__	12:__	1:__	2:__	3:__	4:__	5:__	6:__	7:__	8:__	9:__	10:__	11:__
Blood Sugar																								
Grams of Carb																								
Insulin for Carb																								
Insulin to Correct																								
Total Dose																								
Lantus Dose																								
Ketones																								
Date	12:__	1:__	2:__	3:__	4:__	5:__	6:__	7:__	8:__	9:__	10:__	11:__	12:__	1:__	2:__	3:__	4:__	5:__	6:__	7:__	8:__	9:__	10:__	11:__
Blood Sugar																								
Grams of Carb																								
Insulin for Carb																								
Insulin to Correct																								
Total Dose																								
Lantus Dose																								
Ketones																								

Name: _____ DOB: _____ Telephone # _____ Date: _____

Notes about highs/lows: _____

Figure 1 Sample log sheet for recording insulin and carbohydrate intake.
(Courtesy Maine Medical Partners Pediatric Specialty Group.)

too low to correct the high blood sugar. So either way, your child's blood glucose probably won't get to a healthy level unless you test first.

2. The second thing to consider is whether the child is about to eat (or has just eaten, in some cases) any food containing carbohydrates. If so, you need to determine how much carbohydrate is in the food. We give more details about carbohydrates in Questions 56 and 57, but for now it's essential that you recognize that calculating bolus insulin doses is in part related to the child's current blood sugar, and in part related to the quantity of carbohydrates consumed in each meal or snack.

3. Once you've ascertained the child's current blood glucose level and the amount of carbs in the food, the third variable to consider is how long it's been since your child last had insulin. Insulin has a fairly specific length of duration in the body, and it's important to take into account any insulin currently "on board" before you add more. This is a crucial but often overlooked factor, and it's the primary cause of insulin "stacking" that leads to low blood sugars, particularly at night (see Question 36).

4. And finally, the last factor to consider is the overall environment in which you're giving insulin. Is your child sick or feverish? Is the child about to undertake (or in the middle of) vigorous activity, such as sports or another form of exercise? Is the weather warm or cold? All of these factors might influence how your child responds to insulin, so you would adjust by increasing or decreasing the dose, depending on how your child has responded to them in the past (this is why it's so important to keep records—you won't remember your child's past responses unless you do!)

Keeping all of this in mind, the method for calculating a dose of insulin looks something like the algorithm shown in **Figure 2**.

We'd like to emphasize once more that it's okay to stray from the exact dosage recommended by your calculations if circumstances warrant it. If your child has been trending low or high for a day or 2, parents should absolutely try to compensate for these trends by giving less or more insulin. You will likely be hesitant to do this at first because you fear over- or under-dosing your child, but as time passes, you'll get a better "feel" for what your child really needs and learn to trust your instincts.

It's okay to stray from the exact dosage if circumstances warrant it.

Your diabetes educator will offer you advice on how to develop this understanding, but there are also a multitude of books, web sites, and internet communities full of people who can help you learn. We highly recommend that you learn from people who have been there before you by joining one of the various online communities for people with Type 1 diabetes.

34. Do I give my child insulin before the meal, or after? How long before or after should I give it?

Most of the time, bolus insulin is given before the meal. Studies of children who inject 30 minutes before versus 5 minutes after eating have shown that overall blood glucose control is better when insulin is injected before the meal, not during or after. As long as you have a general sense of how much your child is likely to eat, there is no reason to wait, and giving insulin before a meal allows it to better mimic the action of the insulin a functioning pancreas would release. It does mean, however, that

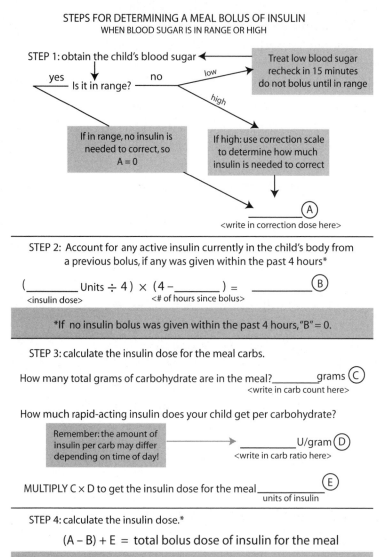

STEPS FOR DETERMINING A MEAL BOLUS OF INSULIN
WHEN BLOOD SUGAR IS IN RANGE OR HIGH

STEP 1: obtain the child's blood sugar

Treat low blood sugar
recheck in 15 minutes
do not bolus until in range

yes   no   low

Is it in range?   high

If in range, no insulin is
needed to correct, so
A = 0

If high: use correction scale
to determine how much
insulin is needed to correct

_____ (A)

STEP 2: Account for any active insulin currently in the child's body from
a previous bolus, if any was given within the past 4 hours*

(_____ Units ÷ 4) × (4 – _____) = _____ (B)
<insulin dose>   <# of hours since bolus>

*If no insulin bolus was given within the past 4 hours, "B" = 0.

STEP 3: calculate the insulin dose for the meal carbs.

How many total grams of carbohydrate are in the meal? _____ grams (C)

How much rapid-acting insulin does your child get per carbohydrate?

Remember: the amount of
insulin per carb may differ
depending on time of day!   _____ U/gram (D)

MULTIPLY C × D to get the insulin dose for the meal _____ (E)
units of insulin

STEP 4: calculate the insulin dose.*

(A – B) + E = total bolus dose of insulin for the meal

*If (A – B) is a negative number, then there is active insulin still available
to correct the high blood sugar and the meal bolus dose = E

Figure 2 Steps for determining a meal bolus of insulin when blood sugar is in range or high. This decision tree represents the sequence of steps needed to calculate how much rapid-acting insulin is required to cover carbohydrates a child consumes in a meal. It takes into account insulin that has already been given in a prior bolus, as well as insulin needed to correct a high blood sugar reading. Keep in mind that if the child has eaten fairly recently (within 2 ½ to 3 hours), he or she already may have insulin on board to bring a high blood sugar back into range (see Question 36 on how to avoid "stacking" insulin). However, this fairly simplified drawing doesn't account for many other factors affecting a dose of insulin, such as planned activity levels, weather or temperature, illness, and so forth. Parents should work with their diabetes educators and clinicians to determine how to adjust bolus doses of insulin up or down as needed to account for such factors.

you have to keep after your child to finish *everything* you offer, because otherwise the excess insulin will bring the child's blood sugar down too low. So be sure you know your child's appetite and food preferences before you go ahead and dose!

How long before the meal you give insulin depends in large part on your child's current blood sugar. It takes about 15 minutes for injected rapid-acting insulin to start bringing blood sugar down, and 1½ to 2½ hours for it to reach peak activity. So if your child's blood sugar is relatively high before the meal—say, in the top half of the target range—you could comfortably give the insulin dose for what you plan to serve 15 minutes (or even 30 minutes) before you expect your child to start eating, because it won't bring the child's blood glucose down into "low" territory prior to the meal. On the other hand, if your child's blood sugar is at the low end of the ideal range before dinner, you might want to hold off on giving the insulin till just before he or she starts to eat, so that the food has a chance to start bringing the blood sugar up a bit before the insulin starts bringing it back down. Your endocrinologist should give you a chart telling you when to give mealtime insulin injections depending on blood sugar levels.

Another factor that may affect when you give insulin is the **glycemic index** of the food you're giving. We explain this concept in Question 53, but as a general rule, food with a high glycemic index breaks down to glucose faster and causes a "spike" in blood sugar, so if you're giving your child food that fits this description (simple carbs such as juice or crackers for example), you'll want to give the insulin a little earlier even if the blood glucose level is in the lower part of the range (but not if it's out of range and low!).

Glycemic index

A measure of the rate at which certain foods cause blood glucose to rise.

The exception to this rule is in children whose eating patterns are unpredictable, such as toddlers and infants. With such young children, you can't really be sure how much they're going to eat in a sitting—or if they're going to eat at all, sometimes! So in these cases, it's better to wait to see how much they actually consume, *then* give sufficient insulin to account for what their carb intake amounts to. The drawback to this strategy is that it allows the carb breakdown into glucose to get a "head start" on the insulin, so the blood sugars after the meal might be considerably higher than they would be if the insulin were given in advance of the food. However, that possibility is better than the opposite—that insulin will be administered but the carbs won't get eaten, and the child then needs either an emergency dose of juice or candy or a glucagon shot when the insulin finds nothing to work with in the bloodstream. You can also split the dose, giving part of the dose at the beginning and the rest after the meal is finished; it requires you to pay closer attention and not get distracted, but it will help to keep the child's blood sugar from going too high.

Elizabeth's comment:

Eric was only 18 months when he was diagnosed, and already a fairly picky eater. I couldn't tell you how much he was going to eat at a sitting if my life depended on it. So we got used to "guesstimating" how much he'd eaten and giving him insulin after he ate—and it did mean that his blood sugars after a meal went up higher, and kept his A1c values pretty high too. As he got older, I got a better sense of what I could expect him to eat and started giving him the insulin earlier in the meal—sometimes, I'd give him half of it when he sat down at his plate, wait to make sure he finished, then give him the other half, just to keep his sugars from going quite so high. Or, if he acted very hungry and the food was something I knew he liked, I'd give it all to him up front and keep my fingers crossed that he finished (and if he didn't, I'd wait an hour or so and then give him a little bit of juice to take care of the insulin that was still in his system). Little by little, we're working toward giving him the insulin ahead of his food.

35. What is the "honeymoon" phase, and how do I know if my child's in it? If my child's in the honeymoon phase, can I stop giving her insulin?

The honeymoon phase may last weeks, months, or even years.

When a child is diagnosed with Type 1 diabetes and started on insulin therapy, many times there is an effect that clinicians refer to as the **honeymoon**. During this phase, the child's pancreas starts producing insulin again, although it's usually only a small amount. Why this occurs isn't quite clear, but it may last weeks, months, or even years before the remaining beta cells are finally overcome by the autoimmune activity.

Honeymoon

A period of time post-diagnosis when beta cells in the pancreas resume producing some insulin.

Parents discover that their child is in honeymoon by the fact that normal doses of insulin can frequently send the child low. If you find yourself repeatedly treating lows or cutting back on doses to avoid lows, chances are good that your child is in honeymoon, particularly if you are still in the first year after diagnosis (honeymoons do happen later than this, but it's not as common). The honeymoon phase is marked by low insulin requirements and stable, near-normal blood glucose levels, so it's welcomed by most parents as a reprieve from intensive management of diabetes. But the need for added insulin does not end, because the pancreatic cells are not able to resume full activity—they are simply an adjunct to the insulin you provide through injections.

The analogy with marriage is accurate because sooner or later, the honeymoon does end, and when it ends, a lifelong relationship between the person with diabetes and their insulin requirements begins. As any newlywed soon discovers, once the honeymoon ends, the work at maintaining this relationship must be taken seriously and given great effort daily if it's to remain healthy for life.

36. What is meant by "stacking" insulin, and how do I avoid it?

"Stacking" insulin is the term used to refer to doses of insulin that overlap, causing an unexpected drop in blood sugar. Usually, **stacking** is a result of failing to take into account insulin that was injected at an earlier time that may not yet have peaked in its activity.

Stacking

Overlapping doses of insulin that cause low blood sugar levels.

Here's a pretty common scenario in which stacking occurs. Let's say your daughter wakes up with a slightly high blood sugar. She immediately has a huge breakfast of orange juice, sausage, pancakes, and syrup. You give her the correct bolus dose for the inordinately high number of carbs she has on her plate, plus additional insulin to correct the high blood sugar. You watch as she gulps down the orange juice first before attacking the pancakes and sausage (and you make sure she eats it all), and then you send her out to play when she's done. An hour or so later, she comes back into the house and says she's hungry again—she wants a snack. You take her blood sugar and find it to be 30 points higher than the upper limit of her target range, so you give her a correction dose along with the dose needed to account for her carbohydrate intake, feed her the snack she has asked for, and send her back out. Two and a half hours after that, she comes in for lunch looking pale and shaky; you test her and find that she's low.

In this case, the mistake was giving the child the second correction dose upon finding her to be high *less than 2 hours after she had been given her initial dose.* The meal she ate had probably just finished going through her system into her bloodstream, but the insulin she'd taken hadn't yet reached its peak activity, so there was plenty of active insulin still in her body to bring the blood sugar down—and a correction really wasn't needed. By giving her the snack, however, the hypoglycemic response that you'd expect when too much insulin was given was delayed, because the excess insulin in her system went right to work on the new set of carbs. At the same time, though, the insulin dose given to cover those carbs got "stacked" on top of what was already there. Once the snack was through her system, there was nothing left for the now-peaking snack-time insulin to work on, and the child became hypoglycemic.

Stacking is best avoided by keeping good records about when insulin is delivered and calculating what remains of the most recent dose before you deliver a new dose. If you know, for instance, that your daughter had her first dose of insulin at 8 AM and that her insulin has a 4-hour duration of action, then you can assume that at 9 AM (1 hour after the injection), she still has about three-quarters of the original dose in her system, and at 10 AM, she still has about one-half of the original dose on board. You therefore wouldn't want to offer any insulin beyond what's needed to take care of any additional food she eats until at least 11:00 AM, 3 hours after the initial dose of insulin was given, because by that point, most of it has gone out of her system and it is past its peak activity.

One rule of thumb to avoid stacking is to only correct highs that are recorded 2½ to 3 hours after a meal. If you have reason to believe that you might overcorrect, use the night-time correction scale, which is usually a little less aggressive. For example, if you find a high blood sugar in your daughter during the first 15 minutes of a soccer game, you know that her excitement and adrenaline are contributing to the high blood sugar, but also that her activity should bring it down over time. In this instance, it's best to give her a correction, but you probably should either use the night-time scale or simply guesstimate how much to reduce the dose based on prior experience.

37. What is an insulin pump?

An insulin pump is a mechanical device for delivering insulin. It's not an artificial pancreas (which is the misconception some people have about it until they learn more). Contrary to many parents' expectations, it doesn't actually do the job of managing diabetes by itself—parents still have to count carbs and take regular blood sugar readings. In essence, it's not much more than a mechanical syringe, but with three important differences: first, because it is able to give insulin in extremely small, targeted amounts, it allows for a much finer and more controlled insulin delivery than can be achieved with syringes; second, it allows the wearer to make adjustments in the amount of basal insulin delivered at any given time, something a syringe can't do; and third, it keeps track of how much insulin has been delivered and is still active in the child's system.

Here's how they operate. The pump's computer is programmed with the wearer's correction factor and basal and bolus ratios, which can be altered according to time of day so that if your child's insulin needs tend to be higher at certain times of day or night, the pump will supply insulin accordingly. The insulin is delivered in amounts as small as 0.05 units/hour via a **cannula** that is inserted using a needle that is either guided manually under the skin, or injected using a mechanical device (after numbing the site with **lidocaine** cream in either case). The cannula and the port attached to it are generally referred to as the **insertion site** or sometimes just called "the site"—so if your diabetes team tells you to "change the site," they're referring to the cannula and port combo. The port itself clips either to an **infusion set**, consisting of a small needle with a plastic clip on the end of long plastic tube about half a millimeter in diameter that connects to the insulin reservoir, or, in the case of self-contained pumps such as the Omnipod, directly into the pump itself. The insertion site and infusion set are changed every 2 to 3 days to avoid irritation or infection of the skin and to assure continued accurate delivery of insulin.

When a child is wearing an insulin pump, the pump will continuously deliver the basal insulin at the rate that has been programmed into it, but bolus insulin will need to be programmed into the pump manually. Your diabetes educator will help you to program in the bolus ratios based on what your child needs, and will also program the pump with the insulin's activity duration so it can calculate the amount of insulin remaining from any previous doses.

Delivering a bolus dose of insulin with a pump goes something like this. First, the child's blood sugar is taken; depending on the meter and pump capabilities, the reading is then either transmitted to the pump automatically or it is manually entered into the pump's computer. The pump then prompts the user to put in the

Cannula

A very fine plastic tube inserted under the skin to deliver insulin.

Lidocaine

A common numbing cream.

Insertion site

The needle, adhesive, port, and cannula combination that is used to infuse insulin under the skin when using an insulin pump.

Infusion set

The clip and tubing that connects the insulin reservoir of an insulin pump to the insertion site where the cannula has been inserted under the skin.

number of carbs in the meal, and once it has this number, the pump computer takes into account the blood sugar level, the carbs to be covered, and any insulin previously administered by the pump to calculate an appropriate bolus dose. The pump then recommends a bolus dose and asks the pump user whether that dose should be delivered.

It's important to understand that the pump does not automatically deliver the dose, but requires the user to make the decision.

It's important to understand that *the pump does not automatically deliver the dose*, but requires the user to make the decision on whether to deliver it, alter it (you can either increase or decrease), or skip it altogether. This is crucial because the pump cannot take into account the user's environment, state of health, or planned activity levels. For example, let's say your child is prone to low blood sugars during hot days, and you've been accustomed to giving the child less insulin when the temperature outside is over 80°. The pump, for all its capabilities, cannot measure the temperature or know how your child will respond, so it's going to be up to you to tell the pump to deliver less insulin than the pump might recommend. Or suppose your child has a cold, and typically runs high when sick; under these circumstances, you might ask the pump to deliver a slightly higher dose. Alternatively, in either of these scenarios, you can set a temporary basal rate that's lower or higher than normal. What it boils down to is that the pump is just a machine, capable of making calculations but not capable of making judgments. So the parent (or the child, if old enough) needs to be able to assess factors such as the weather, the child's overall health, activity levels, and so on to determine whether the dose the pump suggests is correct.

The pump is just a machine, capable of making calculations but not capable of making judgments.

Under some circumstances, pump wearers may use the pump only for bolus delivery and not basal — for example, when a child is extremely uncomfortable wearing the pump at night and there's concern that the child might pull out the insertion site because of this discomfort. In those cases, the child is given long-acting or intermediate-acting insulin at night (see Question 30 about different types of insulin) and only wears the pump during the day, with the basal rate set at 0.0 and bolus doses given as described earlier.

Using a pump is both simpler and more complicated than delivering insulin with a syringe. On the one hand, you don't have to do all the calculations yourself, as that's done by the pump's computer; on the other, you have to learn a whole new set of techniques for handling your child's insulin needs. We'll discuss these pros and cons in the next question.

38. What are the advantages and disadvantages of using an insulin pump versus injections?

You'll likely hear many people singing the praises of insulin pumps, but in truth the advantages and disadvantages are about equal, and it really depends on who's using it whether the pump is a better option than manually delivered insulin. We'll go through the advantages first.

One of the biggest advantages to the pump, especially for very small children, is that it allows for more accurate delivery of insulin (you can give your child as little as .05 units at a time), which means that, assuming that the parent and child are diligent about counting carbs, taking blood sugar readings regularly, and giving correct bolus doses, blood sugar control is generally better. Better blood sugar control, in turn, means less risk of long-term complications, less risk of extreme lows and highs, and less stress for parents and child alike. A pump also offers more flexibility in deciding when and how much to eat, because if the child eats more than originally intended, it's simply a matter of entering the additional carbs into the pump bolus function — you can skip over the blood glucose input and go straight to the carb input function. A pump also allows you or your child to adjust the basal insulin downward — something that isn't possible with long-acting insulin. This is a great advantage when it comes to allowing a child with diabetes to just "be a kid," because if the child wants to participate in sports or gym class, or even simply wants to play hard or run around, he or she can do so without diabetes getting in the way of the fun. With a pump, rather than needing to give the child extra carbs to cover increased activity, a parent can simply decrease the basal rate during or after playtime.

Because the pump computer keeps tabs on how much insulin is left over from the most recent bolus, a pump can provide greater clarity as to how much insulin is currently in your child's bloodstream so you can avoid "stacking" insulin. And best of all, it eliminates the need for multiple injections — particularly valuable for very young children whose parents work, because with minimal training, insulin delivery can be programmed by a daycare provider or teacher without the need for special skills. Many parents of children with Type 1 diabetes feel that a pump offers them more freedom for this reason, among others.

But pumps are not always the better choice, and there are good reasons for some families to prefer manually delivered insulin injections. For one thing, pumps are machines, and machines do occasionally malfunction — and a pump that's dropped on a concrete sidewalk or into a swimming pool (or toilet!) is often a pump that needs to be replaced. And if your child is particularly active or prone to "investigating" mechanical devices, the potential for damage to the device or simple malfunction (a battery or a reservoir pulled out by a curious child, for instance) might be a serious concern. Some parents aren't "gadget-friendly" and have a tough time getting accustomed to how to program the pump for different circumstances—school-age or teenage children often figure it out much more quickly than their parents.

The most serious concern is that unlike injected insulin, where you generally know for certain that the insulin did get delivered, there are several minor reasons why a pump might not deliver the insulin you expect it to—a crimp in the cannula, a cannula that has slipped out from under the skin, and air bubbles in the tubing are a few of the common "nuisance" issues that lead to high blood glucose in pump users. Keep in mind, though, that for a child using a pump, there is no long-acting insulin to act as a "safety net," so if the pump isn't delivering insulin, there is *no* insulin in the child's body *at all*. That means pump users actually have a greater likelihood of ketoacidosis than syringe users. If the child or the parent isn't diligent in monitoring blood sugar levels and watching out for ketones (and we find this frequently happens with teenagers), the "nuisances" described above can turn into DKA and a trip to the hospital! Such problems are less common with syringes, which is why some parents may find that it makes sense to stick with, or even return to, insulin injections.

Pumps also are prohibitively expensive devices for most families when not covered by insurance; fortunately, many insurers will cover them on the theory that the potential for better control of diabetes means lower cost of treatment in the long run. But many insurers won't cover them without evidence that you have tried, and failed, to obtain good control using syringes — another reason to keep good records — and they may balk at covering a pump if your child's blood glucose control is reasonably good with syringes (see our discussion of insurance issues in **Part Six: Other Things Parents Worry About**). In short, they may not pay for it if they feel that changing to pump therapy is about convenience rather than medical necessity.

While fewer injections may be a plus, the pump requires parents and/or the child to learn how to insert a cannula under the skin, which may be more difficult for some. And in general, there's a lot more to learn and understand about the pump's functioning and how it delivers insulin than is required for using syringes, because the pump handles both basal and bolus insulin delivery simultaneously.

There's also the psychological factor to think about. Some children are just not comfortable wearing a pump because they feel "tied down" to this little device that supplies their insulin. The pump is generally worn 24/7, and that can be a little irritating for some kids, particularly children used to being highly active. Moreover, we all know that children tend to pick on kids who are "different," and wearing a pump often draws unwelcome attention to a child with diabetes — attention that they may feel better able to avoid if they're using syringes. So there are many considerations before deciding on whether to use a pump or not.

Ultimately, whether to use a pump or not is a personal choice. Physicians may encourage you to choose a pump because they believe it will provide your child with superior blood glucose control. But your doctor isn't the one who has to learn to use it and live with it — so it's really up to you and your child, if he or she is old enough to make the decision.

Elizabeth's comment:

We started Eric on an insulin pump about 10 months after his diagnosis, after having gotten fairly comfortable giving him diluted insulin with a syringe. At first, it was a mixed bag. On the good side was the fact that using a pump made it a lot easier to cover his carb intake while he's at daycare, because the daycare provider — who just couldn't bring herself to learn how to inject him with a syringe — had no trouble giving him insulin with the pump. And that meant that my husband no longer had to go over to the daycare two or three times a day to provide insulin injections. We also liked the fact that we could give him even miniscule doses of insulin without resorting to diluting the insulin — pretty important in a little guy like Eric who uses such tiny amounts. Putting him on a pump improved our ability to keep his blood sugars in range — and that was a big deal to us because his daily blood sugars and his A1c had been all over the map while he was on diluted insulin given by syringe. So we knew when we started to make the transition that the pump had a great many benefits to offer us and our son.

The downside was the learning curve — in theory the pump sounds easier than syringes, but there's an awful lot you have to learn to make sure the pump functions correctly, and the education process is a little daunting, particularly if you've already gotten the hang of using syringes. You have to think about different things than you do when giving insulin by syringe. On the second night, for instance, we had a problem with air in the line so that Eric wasn't getting the correction doses we were trying to give him — and, during the education process, both my husband and I missed the fact that you're supposed to change the site and re-prime the pump if the blood sugar readings are elevated extremely high. This is a pretty important piece of information that Dr. Olshan wound up passing on at three in the morning after I called him because it was clear to me that something was very wrong! And to make matters worse, our bottle of Lantus had expired that day and I'd thrown it out without thinking about the fact that I didn't have a fresh bottle in the house, so we couldn't switch back to long-acting insulin when the problem continued the next day. We wound up temporarily returning to syringes during a frustrating week that involved several calls to both the clinic and the pump's manufacturer, Medtronic.

With help from Medtronic's technical staff, we solved the air bubble problem, but even then it still wasn't entirely smooth sailing because Eric is so active, we dealt with crimped cannulas on a regular basis. It took us a little while to learn that inserting the cannula in a particular direction helped to prevent that problem. In time, it all sorted itself out. But for about 3 weeks, it was night after sleepless night of checking and adjusting and wondering if it was really going to be worth it. In the end, Eric's A1c values at our first follow-up visit told the story—they went from 8.6 to 8.2 in just 1 month, and by the 1-year anniversary of his transition to pump therapy, they were consistently below 8.

It's clear to us that for all its difficulties, the control we have with the pump is far and away better than what we had with syringes—but our experience has certainly made me realize that putting a child on an insulin pump is a lot more complicated than it seems. It also taught me to never, EVER, let myself get caught without backup supplies, because the minute you're unprepared for a breakdown, that's when it's going to happen.

39. What determines whether my child is eligible for an insulin pump?

From a medical perspective, most children with Type 1 diabetes are eligible for insulin pumps. However, there are other considerations that determine your child's eligibility. First, does your insurance cover insulin pump therapy? Some comprehensive plans do, but many other plans do not, or do so only under very specific circumstances. If your plan restricts coverage of pump therapy devices and supplies, you may need to work with your child's endocrinologist and perhaps an insurance agent to demonstrate to your insurer that your child's health would substantially benefit by use of an insulin pump (which would arguably make pump therapy more cost-effective in the long run). A child whose blood glucose is poorly controlled with syringe treatment—indicated by consistently high A1c results, repeated changes to the insulin regimen with no improvement, or hospital visits for severe hypoglycemia—might be considered a candidate for insulin pump therapy even by insurers who limit access to pumps. (See Questions 85–88 for more on insurance issues.)

The other factor that determines your child's eligibility for pump therapy is the child's tolerance of the pump itself. Some children simply can't accept the physical presence of the pump and associated tubing in close proximity to their bodies. Simply put, it bothers them to the point that they can't focus on anything else. Other children can tolerate the pump itself, but they experience skin irritation related to the cannula, the numbing cream, or the adhesive at the infusion site, which makes wearing the pump intolerable. When pump therapy is being considered, these factors will be tested with a pump filled with saline, not insulin, to make sure the child can tolerate them without putting the child's health at risk. If for some reason the saline trial doesn't work out, pump therapy may not be an option for the child (or, it may have to wait till the child is older, since sensitivities and tolerance levels change over time).

If insurance is the sticking point when it comes to pump therapy, there are organizations that help parents obtain refurbished or even new insulin pumps at no charge and provide low-cost or free supplies in the absence of insurance support. We list these resources in the Appendix.

40. Is it possible to treat diabetes with a pancreas transplant?

It may seem like the most obvious way to handle a problem caused by a pancreas that doesn't function well is to transplant a functioning pancreas into the person with Type 1 diabetes; but the truth is, the side effects and complications related to transplantation are so great that this form of treatment is reserved only for people with very serious diabetic complications, such as kidney failure (the pancreas and kidneys are often transplanted simultaneously). Pancreas transplantation would not save your child from needing lifelong medication, because although insulin injections would no longer be required, anti-rejection medications that suppress the immune system would be necessary to prevent the immune system from attacking the "foreign" pancreas tissue. These immunosuppressive therapies would leave your child vulnerable to a host of opportunistic infections to the point that the health price that the child would pay for having a functional pancreas simply wouldn't be worth it—the child would be sicker, not healthier! Moreover, if the pancreas were to be rejected, your child would end up right back where he or she started—having Type 1 diabetes—with the added complication of having to recover from major surgery. Ultimately, pancreatic transplantation is not the best way to treat Type 1 diabetes except in a few, rare cases.

Researchers have also tried transplanting new beta cells into an individual, rather than transplanting a whole pancreas. There are still certain problems with this approach—mainly how to obtain sufficient beta cells to provide enough insulin (currently, the cells from three adult cadavers are required for one person), and also how to prevent the immune system from simply attacking the transplanted cells. Some researchers are investigating ways to seal off transplanted beta cells from attack by immune cells, and others are working on safer anti-rejection treatments. So while beta cell transplant is a promising concept, it's simply not ready for widespread use in people yet—and given the way new therapies are developed, even should this technique prove workable, it will need to be tested in adults for many years before it will be approved for use in children.

Medical technology is also working toward creating an artificial pancreas by combining the standard insulin pump setup with continuous glucose monitoring and automating it so that it supplies the right amount of insulin to keep blood sugar steady without inducing lows. At this writing, the goal is to have a fully functional prototype ready for FDA review in 2015.

KETONES AND DKA

41. What are ketones?

Ketones are an acidic waste product that is produced when your body burns stored fat for energy. The production of ketones (**ketogenesis**) is normal and not harmful in small amounts, but when ketones are present in large amounts, they can tip the pH of the blood from its normal, slightly alkaline level of 7.35–7.45 to a more acidic level. This development is a very serious threat to health, as too great a departure from the normal blood pH can very quickly lead to dysfunction, even failure, of major organs, particularly the kidneys and heart.

Ketones are a sign that normal glucose transfer from the blood to the cells isn't happening, and the body is turning to fat stores to make up for this problem. They can occur when blood glucose is adequate or high but too little insulin has been delivered to process it. Or they can occur if both glucose and insulin are low (this frequently happens when a child is ill and unable to eat).

42. How and when should I test for ketones?

Parents should test for ketones under the following circumstances:

- When the child's blood glucose is significantly above the normal range, at a level that will be determined by your diabetes team (usually higher than ~240 mg/dL)
- When the child is sick or not eating normally
- When your child appears to have symptoms of diabetic ketoacidosis (see Question 44)

Ketogenesis

Production of ketones.

Ketone testing is something most parents easily overlook because, more often than not, when blood sugars are even very elevated, ketones are negative. This is because ketones develop only when there's a lack of insulin, and not from too much glucose in the blood. For example, if a child with Type 1 diabetes eats a snack that's high in carbohydrates but does not cover it with insulin, he/she will likely have a blood glucose over 300 mg/dL. However, this by itself will rarely produce ketones because the child's long-acting insulin (or basal insulin, if on a pump) provides enough insulin to allow the body to meet its basic energy needs. On the other hand, if the long-acting insulin dose is overlooked (or the pump isn't delivering basal insulin for some reason), and the child goes even 4 hours during the day without eating or taking short-acting insulin, he/she is likely to start developing ketones. Fortunately, high blood glucose is only rarely associated with large ketones—but when it does happen, the consequences can be life threatening! For this reason, whenever there is an unexpected high blood sugar, it is critical that parents check for ketones.

Ketones can also develop when children are chronically low due to illness, so testing for ketones during a period of sickness is also helpful. Ketones are also more likely to show up in pump users who have both basal and bolus insulin delivered via pump, because if the pump's delivery of insulin fails for any reason, it means the child is without any source of background insulin—and ketones will start to show up within 2–4 hours if the problem isn't discovered and corrected.

For older children (4 years and up, or younger if potty trained), you probably will be instructed to test with urine ketone strips. Your child can either urinate directly onto the strip or into a cup that you can then use to dip the strip into. For children still in diapers, a cotton ball placed in the diaper can help you obtain a sample, or you can use a blood ketone meter, which tests in much the same way a blood glucose meter does. Be aware, though, that blood ketone meters and the strips that go with them are considerably more expensive than urine ketone strips, so if you're paying out-of-pocket, the cost difference might become an incentive to potty-train your child sooner!

43. What should I do if my child has high ketones?

Ketones only occur when the child is burning fat for energy, and that usually only happens when the child doesn't have enough insulin on board to process glucose. When the child's blood glucose is high, the obvious solution to ketones is to give the child insulin so that the glucose already in the blood can be ushered into the cells so that fat-burning for energy can stop.

If your child uses an insulin pump and has ketones, give the correction dose by syringe, not via the pump. Then check to make sure the pump is functioning correctly, and change the insertion site if necessary.

If your child gets insulin via syringes, you should give your child a correction dose for the high blood sugar immediately, and follow whatever other instructions your diabetes team gave you regarding handling ketones. If your child is on a pump, it's quite possible that the ketones are a symptom of a crimped cannula or an air bubble in the line, so give the insulin dose via syringe, not via the pump. Once you've given your child insulin with the syringe, you can check to make sure the pump is working properly and change the child's insertion site if necessary.

Where it gets complicated is if your child's blood sugar is low, because the adding insulin will only make the child's blood sugar lower—perhaps dangerously low.

That means that once you've given the insulin, you need to feed your child sufficient carbohydrates to keep the blood glucose level in the normal range. If your child has low blood sugar because of illness, this can be a problem — sick children aren't likely to want to eat much, and if the child vomits up what you offer, it complicates matters still more. A situation like this definitely warrants a call to your diabetes clinic for advice. (For more on handling sick days, see **Part Four: Sick Days**.)

> **TIP FOR PUMP USERS**
>
> If you give your child a correction with a syringe, you may want to keep the pump's computer up-to-date on how much insulin is in your child's system. To do this, disconnect the pump from the insertion site port, program the bolus dose you gave by syringe into the pump's computer, and hold the tubing over the sink while the insulin drips out — that way, the pump will record the bolus dose but you will be certain your child got the insulin. Then, change the insertion site and check the infusion set's tubing for bubbles. If any are present, either prime them out or fill a new reservoir before reattaching the infusion set to the port.

If your child is not sick, you can give him or her a dose of insulin (by syringe — again, do not use a pump to deliver insulin to a child with ketones until you've changed the insertion site) followed by high-carb sweets like chocolate syrup or candy that will prevent hypoglycemia. Don't be afraid to go overboard on the carbs in this case, because a high can be corrected; it's more important at this point to avoid a severe low, and to stop fat-burning and get rid of the ketones.

If the child *is* sick, the carbohydrates to turn to are simple carbs that are easily digestible and not likely to produce nausea or vomiting — gingerale, Gatorade, and similar drinks are generally recommended, because ketones often go hand-in-hand with dehydration. Especially if the child has a stomach bug, you need to hold off on giving the child insulin until you're sure that at least some of the carbohydrate you gave is going to stay down. Once your child's blood sugar has risen above the upper limit, you can go ahead and correct a little at a time using your child's night time correction scale. Do not give one large dose of insulin, because if the child vomits up the food at any point, you will have more insulin on board than you have carbohydrates (with limited likelihood of getting more carbs in), and your child is likely to develop hypoglycemia. This situation is the most concerning and would be a good reason to call your diabetes team or consider taking your child to an emergency department.

44. What is diabetic ketoacidosis?

Diabetic keto-acidosis (DKA)

A complication of diabetes that occurs when ketones build up in the bloodstream sufficiently to lower blood pH below its normal level of about 7.35. DKA can be life-threatening if untreated.

Diabetic ketoacidosis (DKA) is a condition that occurs when ketones build up in the blood stream sufficiently to start to alter the normal pH of the blood, making it more acidic than normal. Blood pH generally stays between 7.35 and 7.45 (a slightly alkaline level), and anything that brings it outside that range can cause very serious health complications in a very short time.

As we mentioned in Questions 41 and 44, ketones are a byproduct of burning fat for fuel in the absence of insulin; ketoacidosis develops after this lack of insulin is prolonged. Many parents will have encountered DKA at the time their child was diagnosed, since some children don't get diagnosed with Type 1 diabetes until they show significant symptoms of the disease—at which point can occur. But aside from the time of diagnosis, DKA most often occurs in children as a result of lack of sufficient insulin and can be related to an underlying infection, such as influenza, pneumonia, or even urinary tract infections. And it's important for parents to understand that this can happen even in children who normally have excellent blood glucose control, because infections affect the cells' need for insulin—sometimes dramatically.

In older children, particularly teenagers, DKA can also develop from a desire to lose weight. Adolescents with Type 1 diabetes learn pretty quickly that they can slim down rapidly (without starving themselves like their healthy peers) by simply not using insulin when they eat. This strategy, which is often (unofficially) referred to as "diabulimia," is particularly common in teens who already have an eating disorder such as anorexia or bulimia, but adolescent girls with Type 1 diabetes also appear to be especially prone to eating disorders—so it's something of a chicken-and-egg question as to which came first. As a result, parents of teens and pre-teens with Type 1 diabetes need to be aware that their child could develop DKA for social or emotional reasons rather than because of ill health, and be on the lookout for signs that your child isn't managing her (or his) diabetes properly as well as watching for symptoms of DKA (described in Question 45).

Without sending parents into a panic, we would like to make the point that *DKA is a life-threatening condition.* Unless it is treated relatively quickly, DKA will cause coma and death, so it's not something to take lightly. But the best treatment for DKA is preventing it from happening in the first place, which is why we stress that parents need to strive for good control of the child's blood glucose levels, regularly monitor blood glucose, and know when to check ketone levels.

The best treatment for DKA is preventing it from happening in the first place!

45. What are the symptoms of DKA? How is DKA treated?

Diabetic ketoacidosis symptoms likely resemble the very symptoms that caused you to bring your child to the doctor at the time you received the diabetes diagnosis. They include:

- Excessive thirst
- Frequent urination
- Nausea and vomiting
- Abdominal pain
- Loss of appetite
- Weakness or fatigue
- Confusion or dizziness
- A general ill appearance
- Dry skin
- Dry mouth
- Increased heart rate
- Shortness of breath
- Increased rate of breathing
- Fruity-scented breath

Dehydration is particularly common in DKA because the body excretes greater quantities of fluids driven by the high blood sugar—this is why thirst and frequent urination are the most obvious symptoms that something is amiss. If you test for ketones using either urine or blood ketone strips, you'll also see high levels upon testing.

Treatment of DKA requires a trip to the hospital.

Treatment of DKA requires a trip to the hospital. Typically, your child will be given intravenous fluids to combat the dehydration and, if the child's blood glucose level is low, a glucose drip to raise glucose levels sufficiently so that insulin can be given (if the blood glucose levels are already above 240 mg/dL, insulin can and should be given right away—before you head out to the hospital, if possible). Your child's electrolyte levels are likely to be out of balance, requiring intravenous fluids. Depending on whether there are other health issues that sometimes accompany severe ketoacidosis (swelling of the brain being the most serious complication that can occur more often in children), other treatment options might also be initiated.

EMERGENCY CARE

46. What do I do if my child has a severe low glucose reading or shows signs of "crashing"?

For a parent of a newly diagnosed child, it's hard to know what's truly a hypoglycemic emergency and what's a minor inconvenience. So it's worth defining what constitutes a mild concern, what's a moderate concern, and what's very serious when it comes to hypoglycemia.

When a child's blood glucose is slightly below the lower limit of the target range, it's generally not a major issue—the lower limit is usually set about 5–30 points higher than what would be considered truly low (about 80 mg/dL is a normal, pre-breakfast blood glucose level) so that parents can act before the child becomes truly hypoglycemic and starts experiencing symptoms. So a blood sugar reading of 70 to 100 is still within the "safe zone", and a quick snack of 15 carbs will ensure that an emergency can be avoided—although keep in mind that there is a margin of error in all blood glucose meters, so if your child has symptoms of low blood sugar when the meter says he or she is above 70, you should be sure you wash the child's hand and repeat the test. Remember, problems other than low blood sugar can sometimes produce similar symptoms, such as stress, anxiety, or allergic reactions.

It's also a good idea to do this if you've seen a dramatic drop in blood glucose readings over a relatively short time—100 points over half an hour or so—because if the blood sugar is dropping that fast, hypoglycemia might not be far behind, assuming there's still active insulin on board. Such rapid-onset lows characterized by the sudden development of hypoglycemic symptoms are commonly called "crashes". Take a look at how long it's been since the last bolus, and if the bolus insulin hasn't yet peaked or is in the process of peaking (that is, it's been 2 to 3 hours since it was delivered) and your child is nearing the lower part of the target range, offer 10 to 15 carbs just to be safe.

Blood glucose readings between 60 and 70 are a greater cause for concern. In this range, your child may be mildly hypoglycemic, may experience symptoms of dizziness, shakiness, or lethargy, and needs 15 grams of fast-acting carbohydrate (a 4 oz juice box, for instance) to restore normal blood sugar. But as long as you have a fast-acting carbohydrate handy (juice, soda, or candy such as Smarties, Skittles, jelly beans, or some similar high-sugar, low fat variety), even this isn't an emergency—although if you can't get some fast-acting carbs into the child, it could quickly become one. You will learn fairly soon in your diabetes journey, if you haven't already, that it's essential to *always* keep some form of carbohydrate that your child can be counted on to eat or drink close at hand—and it's likely that one of these moderate hypoglycemic episodes will be the reason you learn why preparedness is key. Your child's situation becomes urgent when the blood glucose level slips below 60, and anywhere below 50 has the potential to become an emergency. Your most important action at this point is to *not panic*, even if your child begins to go extremely low (into the 40s, 30s, or 20s), loses consciousness, has a seizure, or all of the above.

It's essential to always keep some form of carbohydrate close at hand for hypoglycemic episodes.

That last paragraph is probably pretty scary to contemplate if you're new to Type 1 diabetes, so take a moment to breathe and relax if you find yourself getting tense. These frightening possibilities may happen to even the most experienced parent, but they can be overcome with a little planning and mental rehearsal. It is very important that you be prepared to handle severe hypoglycemia, because sooner or later it *will* happen.

When your child is in a state of severe hypoglycemia, and particularly if the child is convulsing or unconscious, the most important treatment is to get his or her blood sugar up *immediately*. If the child is responsive and cooperative, you can still give juice, soda, chocolate or maple syrup, or a tube of cake gel (we don't advise solids like candy because of the danger of choking should the child start to convulse). But if the child won't or can't consume anything, or if the child is having a seizure, it's best to use the glucagon kit (described in Question 48) supplied by your endocrinologist. *If you are at all uncertain about whether you can get carbs into your child fast when the child is severely hypoglycemic, use the kit immediately.*

In severe hypoglycemia, the most important treatment is to get the child's blood sugar up immediately!

47. If my child is hypoglycemic but won't drink juice, how do I quickly improve his blood sugar?

There is little more frustrating and frightening to a parent than realizing that the child desperately needs some carbohydrate, only to have the child refuse to drink the juice you offer! In such situations, there are a few rules of thumb to live by. First, *do not panic or become angry with your child*. Becoming agitated will only make your child's emotional state worse—and bear in mind that your child's emotional state is a result of poor brain function because of the low blood glucose. Your child is not being deliberately defiant or disobedient and, though you may feel frustrated and angry, remember that these feelings are misplaced. Set them aside, and concentrate on taking care of your child.

Second, make sure that you have several options to offer the child so that you can swap the first choice quick-acting carb (usually juice or candy) for something more appealing should your child object. Although your first choice should be something that works fast, your second should be something you know your child likes a lot—even if you think that your first choice would be far better for the child's blood glucose at this given moment. For example, if your child likes chocolate milk better than juice, offer the juice first, but quickly substitute the milk if the child fights you about drinking the juice. Though this seems counterintuitive, remember that the important thing is to treat the low blood sugar quickly, and if your child is refusing the juice, then no treatment is underway—and a slower-acting carb like chocolate milk is better than no carb at all. It may be that once your child has gotten a little bit of a boost from the milk, you can successfully offer juice should it still be needed. Also, if the child refuses the first source of quick-acting carbs you offer, patiently continue to offer your child alternative sources of carbohydrates while explaining in simple terms that he or she will feel better by taking the juice, candy, syrup, cake gel, glucose tablets, or whatever it is you're offering.

Of course, if your child is completely opposed to eating or drinking *anything*, there's a limit to how long you should try to coax and persuade, particularly if the blood glucose measured extremely low (less than 50). One option in this situation is to take a small tube of cake gel and squirt it into your child's mouth between the cheek and gum, where the sugars can be absorbed through the membranes of the mouth. This technique can also be used with juice boxes that come with a straw; you can slip the straw into the mouth between cheek and gums and squeeze the box so that juice squirts up through the straw into where it can be absorbed directly through the membranes. Bear in mind that if the child is really agitated, he or she might bite down on the straw and prevent juice from flowing, so you want to get it *in front of* your child's teeth next to the lining of the cheek. Again, once a little bit of the sugar is absorbed, your child may realize that it feels good to drink the juice and start drinking it voluntarily.

However, if even this doesn't work, remember that you can always use the glucagon kit (described in Question 48) to quickly raise blood sugar in an emergency. Although most parents think of this kit as a last resort and will do anything to avoid using it, if your child is unwilling or unable to take any carbohydrate at all, using a glucagon injection is surely better than nothing!

Elizabeth's comment:

It can be pretty frightening when you find your child's blood glucose at a very low level, and then when you offer a juice box and get a screaming tantrum, that's absolutely terrifying! And if you're like me, panic sometimes triggers anger—in the first few months after his diagnosis, I would get so frightened that his refusal was going to lead to seizures or worse, that I got mad at him for refusing the thing that I knew would prevent that. I'll confess that there were a couple of times when I tried to force my son to drink juice he didn't want because I was so desperate to get his blood glucose up, but all that did was make him choke (and once he just puked the juice back up because he was so upset—which only made the whole thing that much worse!) Over time, I've learned to control my panic and stay calm, and to take the time to comfort my son before offering him various options. I've found that as long as I'm patient, no matter how bad he feels, he'll take some carbohydrate after a little while ... though sometimes those few minutes seem like eons to me! And he's less likely to start fighting me if I remain relaxed and patient from the beginning.

48. What is a glucagon kit? How and when do I use it?

Glucagon

A pancreatic hormone that stops insulin from transferring glucose into the cells.

Glucagon is a pancreatic hormone that is secreted by the pancreatic alpha cells (as opposed to the beta cells that secrete insulin). It's kind of like an "anti-insulin" in that it gets released when blood sugar falls too low, rather than rising too high, and its job is to induce the liver to release stored glucose (glycogen) into the bloodstream and raise blood sugar. You may recall that insulin's job is the opposite: It removes glucose from the blood and transfers it into the cells. This prevents blood sugar from continuing to decrease in the absence of food and is one of the mechanisms that allows people without diabetes to maintain stable blood sugar even when fasting.

Glucagon kit

A pre-loaded emergency kit containing a syringe, saline, and powdered glucagon used to treat extreme low blood sugars.

Because it has the ability to raise blood sugar levels very rapidly, glucagon is extremely valuable as a "rescue" treatment for severe hypoglycemia. At the time of your child's initial diagnosis, you should have been given or prescribed a **glucagon kit** similar to the one shown in **Figure 3**. This kit contains a syringe pre-filled with a diluting solution and a small vial containing glucagon, in the form of a fine white powder, which are stored together in a bright orange or red box. There are two kits widely

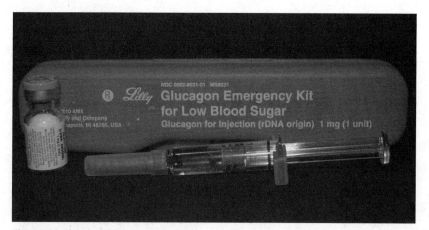

Figure 3 Glucagon kit. (Photo by E. Platt)

available in the United States—one produced by Novo Nordisk (orange box) and the other by Eli Lilly (red box). Both work in the same manner and are equally effective.

If you read the manufacturer's "indications for use" instructions on the flyer accompanying the kit, you'll see that they recommend use of a glucagon kit as a treatment for severe hypoglycemia under the following circumstances:

a. If your child is unable to eat or drink something containing sugar

b. If your child repeatedly eats or drinks something sugary but blood glucose levels remain low

c. If your child becomes unconscious due to low blood sugar and is therefore unable to swallow

d. If your child is having seizures or convulsions, making it dangerous to offer something to eat or drink because of the risk of choking

To use a glucagon kit, you will insert the syringe needle into the vial of powder and push the plunger on the needle so that the diluting solution is added to the powder. Mix the powder well with the solution by gently shaking the vial, then withdraw the dose you need from the vial into the syringe and inject it into your child—any site will do, as long as it's away from the face or major arteries and veins (thigh, butt, or upper arm are usually the best choices). In general, a half dose (500 mg for a Lilly glucagon kit; 0.5 mL for a Novo Nordisk kit) is used for children under 50 pounds, and a full dose (1,000 mg/1.0 mL) for children over 50 pounds. *If you are uncertain of your child's weight, give a full dose—you cannot overdose your child on glucagon.* A full dose will not harm your child, but an insufficient dose might not solve the problem. When hypoglycemia is severe, it's better to give too much than too little. Your child's blood sugar should rebound quite rapidly—within 10 to 15 minutes.

You cannot overdose your child on glucagon, so give a full dose if you're not certain of your child's weight.

Because glucagon can sometimes cause vomiting, try to offer the child a container so that the discomfort of low blood sugar isn't compounded by vomiting on his or her own clothing. And if the child is unconscious, be sure he or she is lying on a flat surface on one side, to avoid choking if vomiting occurs.

You might be wondering where in all this you're supposed to dial 9-1-1—after all, this *is* an emergency, right? Shouldn't you call emergency services before messing around with the glucagon kit? You may be surprised to learn that dialing 9-1-1 in this case is the wrong thing to do because it won't help your child nearly as much, or as quickly, as injecting glucagon. In fact, getting an EMT involved *before* injecting glucagon could cause more harm than good, because once an EMT, paramedic, or doctor takes over your child's care, you may not be permitted to inject the glucagon, and a doctor's authorization may be required to proceed with the injection—a waste of precious time. If your child is unconscious or convulsing and you are frightened enough to want to summon an ambulance, by all means do so—*AFTER* you have injected the glucagon!

Elizabeth's comment:

At the end of our four-day stay in the pediatric ward the week Eric was diagnosed, Dr. Olshan explained how to use the glucagon kit, and of course I asked at what point we called 9-1-1. I was shocked by his answer: "Don't. Emergency service people don't have any better idea of what do to for your child than you do, and what's worse, they may prevent you from giving him a glucagon shot. You need to understand that you now know a lot about how to treat a diabetes crisis, so it's YOUR job to handle it—and you'll likely do it better than they would."

I was horrified by this at first—how could I, overwhelmed and with only four days of information that I wasn't sure I really understood, be better able to care for my son than trained emergency medical workers? But a few weeks later, Eric had a low blood sugar in a restaurant, and just after we left, he threw up the food and the juice I had given him to bring his blood sugar up. When I tested him after he vomited, I found his blood glucose was 34, but couldn't get him to drink any juice because he started to pass out. So I got out the kit and used it, then took him to the hospital—and by the time I got there, 10 minutes later, his blood sugar was in the 200s and he was perky as could be. The people in the ER listened to my story, asked a few questions, confessed that they didn't know much about it but that he seemed to be fine, then sent us on our way—it was a totally unnecessary and rather pointless visit. From that experience, I came to realize that Dr. Olshan was right... and that it was OK that my husband and I were the first line of defense for our son, because this was something we really COULD handle better than anyone else.

49. How do I know when to take my child to the hospital?

As we mentioned above, most hypoglycemic episodes can and should be handled at home. The time to call 9-1-1 and go to the hospital comes when you've taken all the steps to prevent or reverse hypoglycemia but your child's blood sugar isn't going up, or if your child is unconscious or having a seizure and your efforts to bring up the child's blood sugar don't improve his or her condition. You should also contact your diabetes team's emergency triage services if you suspect your child may have diabetic ketoacidosis—or, if you feel it's an emergency, take your child to the nearest hospital with an emergency department.

Emergency intervention in a hospital is most likely to become necessary when:

- Your child is vomiting and you are unable to keep blood sugar levels in the safe zone because he or she can't keep any food down
- Your child has high ketones, something that also can happen when the child is too ill to eat (even if vomiting isn't an issue) or when the child isn't getting adequate amounts of insulin (missing injections or pump failure)
- Your child has symptoms of diabetic ketoacidosis (see Question 45)

50. What do I do if my child becomes comatose?

Coma is something all parents dread, but it's actually not that common for children to slip into a diabetic coma, even when they have low blood glucose while they're sleeping. But you wouldn't be the first parent to be unable to wake your child in the morning and go into a panic thinking the child is comatose! So the first action you need to take if your child is unresponsive is to make sure your child is *actually comatose* and not simply deeply asleep. Do all the things you'd normally do to wake your child, and if he or she doesn't respond, stop and listen to the child's breathing. Is it fast, faint, and shallow? Then look at your child's color. Is it normal, or pale? Does your child's skin feel cool and clammy? Is he or she sweating profusely? If you answer "yes" to these questions, you may have a comatose child on your hands.

At this point, your first act should be to inject glucagon (see Question 48), even before checking the blood sugar level. Then, within 2 minutes after injecting glucagon, take the child's blood sugar before the glucagon has a chance to bring it up—that will give you an accurate idea as to whether the child was comatose from a low blood sugar, or if the blood sugar is already extremely high (see the next paragraph for what to do if it's high). Bear in mind that if your child's blood glucose is extremely low, the meter may not be able to read it, in which case you'll get an error message or a "LO" indication on your meter. If that happens, check again in a few minutes to see if the injection has brought the blood glucose up to a readable level. If your child doesn't rouse soon after the injection, at this point you should probably call 9-1-1 and take him or her to the hospital.

A coma associated with high blood sugar means there's a strong possibility that DKA is the problem (see Questions 44 and 45). While this is a highly unlikely event (usually, you'll see the signs of DKA long before the child becomes comatose), if it does occur, the child should be given a correction via syringe for the highest blood glucose reading on your correction scale, then taken immediately to the nearest hospital emergency department.

PART THREE

Feeding a Child with Diabetes

Does my child's diet need to change?

Does a child with diabetes have special nutritional needs? Does my child need vitamin supplements?

What is meant by "glycemic index," and how does the glycemic index of food affect my child's blood sugar?

More . . .

51. *Does my child's diet need to change?*

This is one of those questions we could answer both ways: no, it doesn't, and yes, it does.

A child with Type 1 diabetes is able to eat everything anyone else can eat, as long as the child is given adequate insulin to process the carbohydrates in the food. In that respect, you don't need to change your child's diet, because everything you have in your fridge and cupboard is OK for your child to eat (barring a diagnosis of celiac disease or other food-related allergy or sensitivity).

You will find, however, that particular foods or food ingredients affect your child's blood sugar and insulin needs in different ways. You may feel more comfortable giving certain foods less often in order to prevent instability in the child's blood sugars, and substituting others that have less of an impact on insulin use. For example, if your child drank a lot of juice or soft drinks before being diagnosed, you may want to try to change your child's usual beverage to milk or water, both of which have fewer carbs. Both require much less insulin, and neither is likely to shoot your child's blood sugar up the way soft drinks or juice would. Flavored waters and low-carb juices that use sucralose, agave nectar, or stevia leaf are also alternatives. You can even try beverages like iced tea (sugarless) or seltzer. Similarly, if your child is fond of cheese or celery sticks with peanut butter for a snack, you may want to offer these options more often than you would have previously because they represent foods that your child can eat a lot of without needing as much insulin to cover them.

What makes it tricky is that different children respond in different ways to different foods. Even if you give insulin to match the carb count on the label, your child may

WHAT ABOUT BREASTFEEDING?

For toddlers and infants who are breastfed, some endocrinologists advise parents to switch to formula or to bottle-feed pumped breast milk (each ounce of breast milk has about 2 carbs). However, abruptly changing from breast to bottle might be stressful for both the child and the mother on the heels of the diabetes diagnosis. Breastfeeding is as much about bonding and comfort as it is about food, so this may not be in your child's best interest.

If your child is eating solid foods regularly and only nurses for comfort, he or she probably isn't getting more than an ounce or 2 of breast milk at a feeding, so switching to a bottle makes little sense. A little experimenting with a breast pump will let Mom determine by sensation how much milk can be drawn from the breast when it "feels full" or when it doesn't. Or, Mom can simply encourage nursing only at times when the child would normally get a "free" snack of 10–15 carbs not covered by insulin, since 5 ounces of breast milk is about 10 carbs.

A younger infant is more of a challenge, but again, using a breast pump for a few days can give a general sense of how much milk is produced at any given time of day in each breast (they don't always produce the same amount). Use the breast pump at the times your child normally breast-feeds, recording the amount of milk you get from each breast until you've worked out roughly how much you get on average at any given time of day or night. Make sure the breast is completely drained. Then, resume breastfeeding and use the averages you calculated as your carb counts, but pay close attention to your child's blood glucose values 2 hours after each feeding. If they're high or low, your child may be getting a little more or less than you estimated, so adjust your calculations with the next feeding, giving a little bit more (or less) insulin depending on the result you got before. Eventually, you'll get a feel for it if you're persistent.

If all of this is too overwhelming, however, don't feel guilty about switching to a bottle or weaning altogether — but DO offer your child extra cuddling and closeness so the child can still experience the emotional benefits of nursing even if the breast milk itself isn't available.

still go high (or low) unexpectedly, simply because the child's system processes the particular food ingredients more or less efficiently than you might expect. You're going to have to figure out whether there are any specific foods that make your child's blood sugar shoot up (or conversely that keep it relatively stable) by watching what happens after your child eats them.

Keeping track of what your child eats and the insulin requirements and blood sugar response in the hours after the meal is the best way to learn the child's patterns. (You can use a food chart like the one in **Figure 4** as a guide.) Get very familiar with the ingredients on food labels, and try different brands now and then to see if the alternative combination of ingredients affects the child in different ways from your usual brand. Selecting brands with less sugar, high fructose corn syrup, or honey in them is generally a good idea, as all of these sweeteners have a high glycemic index (see Question 53) and tend to push blood sugar higher—but at the same time, be aware that, depending on what other ingredients are in the food, your child may be just fine eating foods with these ingredients. Until you try them, you don't know how your child's blood sugar will respond. Similarly, different preservatives, fillers, or starches may also affect your child's blood sugar in different ways. You'll only find out how *your* child responds to specific ingredients by trial and error. Over time, you'll get a better idea of what foods destabilize your child's blood sugar and be able to limit or avoid them.

As always, we recommend you try to offer a *balanced* diet that includes complex carbohydrates, protein, monosaturated fats, and fiber, with an emphasis on vegetables, fruits, nuts, dairy products, and lean meats—even though we know that's not always easy to do.

Elizabeth's comment:
Eric is still pretty limited in what he's willing to eat, but we've figured out a few things about the foods he prefers. One is that we get more stability if we make sure he gets protein

Breakfast	Time _____	Blood Sugar _____			
Food Offered	Amount (oz/#)	Potential Carbs	Actually Ate	Actual Carbs	Notes

AM Snack	Time _____	Blood Sugar _____			
Food Offered	Amount (oz/#)	Potential Carbs	Actually Ate	Actual Carbs	Notes

Lunch	Time _____	Blood Sugar _____			
Food Offered	Amount (oz/#)	Potential Carbs	Actually Ate	Actual Carbs	Notes

PM Snack	Time _____	Blood Sugar _____			
Food Offered	Amount (oz/#)	Potential Carbs	Actually Ate	Actual Carbs	Notes

Dinner	Time _____	Blood Sugar _____			
Food Offered	Amount (oz/#)	Potential Carbs	Actually Ate	Actual Carbs	Notes

Figure 4 Sample food chart for tracking how a child responds to specific foods.
(Courtesy M. Jolin)

or fiber with his food — it seems to slow down the speed his blood sugar rises after he eats. Another is that dairy foods with a lot of sugar will bring his blood sugar high and keep it there — ice cream and chocolate milk, and to a lesser extent yogurt, are sure ways to get his blood sugars up and keep them up when he's trending low. Before we figured that out, there were times we'd give these to him at meals or snacks and find him way up in the 300s 2 hours later! So we keep the pre-packaged chocolate milk boxes around for when he has overnight lows, and he can have ice cream in the evening if his bedtime blood sugar is below 100, but he generally doesn't get it any other time. What's interesting is that not all brands of chocolate milk affect him the same way — we've used Hershey's, Nesquick, and Horizon Organics brands, and each one is different in its effects. But aside from that, we offer him whole milk, seltzer (weird thing to give a preschooler, but he loves it), and tea instead of juice.

52. Does a child with diabetes have special nutritional needs? Does my child need vitamin supplements?

Children with diabetes have the same nutritional needs as other children, and the decision to give your child vitamin supplements is something you should discuss with your pediatrician.

Children with diabetes have the same nutritional needs as other children, and the decision to give your child vitamin supplements is something you should discuss with your pediatrician. In general, if your child eats a variety of foods including ample fresh fruits and vegetables, fish, eggs, and dairy products, *most* of what he or she needs is probably provided by the food. However, if you and your family eat what's commonly called the "standard American diet" — heavy on starches, meats, dairy, and simple carbs, and light on vegetables, whole grains, and fruit — then it's likely that your child is missing some important vitamins and minerals, particularly the vitamins found in leafy green vegetables. If this is the case, then it may be worth offering your child a vitamin supplement. We don't recommend you use the popular "gummy bear" style supplements because children, especially young children, tend to confuse them with candy.

One vitamin that has received a lot of press in connection to Type 1 diabetes is vitamin D. Studies have shown that many children with Type 1 diabetes are substantially deficient in vitamin D (which, unlike many other vitamins, is made by our skin when it's exposed to the ultraviolet rays in sunlight). Vitamin D has been suggested to prevent or delay many diseases, ranging from cancer to heart disease to autoimmune disorders. Many researchers have suggested that higher levels of vitamin D could prevent or at least slow the development of Type 1 diabetes in at-risk children. Opinions are still mixed on whether vitamin D deficiency contributes to the development of diabetes, but experts agree that at least 70% of children in the U.S., with diabetes or without, do not get enough of it, and this lack may be contributing to long-term health problems.

There are many reasons for this situation, some of which may apply to your child. One is a more sedentary, indoors-focused lifestyle that keeps kids out of the sun. A second, related problem is that concern about the potential for skin cancer due to overexposure to the sun has led people to slather their children with sunblock or cover their skin with hats and jackets. This means that children often don't get sufficient sun exposure to make vitamin D in their skin—which in even the fairest-skinned children can be accomplished in far less time than it takes to burn (10 to 15 minutes for light-skinned individuals). The problem is particularly acute in children living in northern latitudes (north of New York City) because from October to April, the sun is too low in the sky for ultraviolet rays to pass through the atmosphere, so that production of vitamin D in skin is curtailed. Children with olive or dark skin also tend to be more likely to experience deficiency because they need more sun exposure to make vitamin D than light-skinned children.

Your child may have been given a vitamin D test at the time of diagnosis. It's worth asking your endocrinologist if this is the case, and find out what your child's levels were. Anything lower than 30 ng/mL is too low—and some experts believe that levels of 50 ng/mL are needed to prevent disease. If your child's levels are low or marginal, you may want to supplement with vitamin D. Talk to your pediatrician about dosing, but be aware that the usual recommended dose of 400 IU is not going to be sufficient to bring a deficient level up (and your pediatrician may not be aware of the discrepancy). Current recommendations suggest that 1,000–2,000 IU is likely an appropriate amount for adolescents and adults.

If your child is able to swallow tablets, vitamin D pills are cheap and easy to find in pharmacies —vitamin D3 (cholecalciferol) is better absorbed than vitamin D2 (ergocalciferol). If your child isn't able to swallow pills, an easy way to provide vitamin D (if your child is willing) is to give your child cod liver oil—sounds gross, but there's a reason our great-grandparents used this "tonic" on their children! It's rich in both vitamin D and omega-3 fatty acids, both of which have well-known health benefits. It's also sold in different flavors (lemon is particularly popular). If cod liver oil doesn't do it, there are also vitamin D drops available in drug stores from manufacturers such as Gerber or Enfamil, or online from Carlson Labs. These can be added to your child's water or milk, as they're flavorless and colorless.

53. What is meant by "glycemic index" and how does the glycemic index of food affect my child's blood sugar?

In Question 23, we talked about why carbohydrates matter to children with diabetes, and how there are different forms of carbohydrate that break down differently when eaten. But even that isn't the full story. The speed at which carbs are digested and converted to glucose also depends on whether the food also contains protein, fiber, or fats, which can slow the breakdown of the carbohydrates in the food.

The **glycemic index** is a way of measuring how quickly blood sugar rises in response to eating a particular food. It accounts for the full range of elements—the carbohydrate, fats, protein, and fiber—and how they affect food breakdown and absorption. A food with a low glycemic index raises blood sugar slowly and gradually, while a food with a high glycemic index raises blood sugar rapidly. Getting to know the glycemic index of your child's favorite foods can help you determine when to give insulin in relation to the meal so that blood sugar doesn't "spike" (see Question 34) or, alternately, so that the insulin doesn't peak before the food is fully digested. Learning, in general, what foods cause blood sugar to shoot high very rapidly, what foods don't have this effect, and how to pair foods so that blood sugar rises more slowly rather than "spiking" is worth the effort. In our Appendix, we include a number of resources describing glycemic index and a related concept, **glycemic load** (which, simply put, uses the glycemic index of the food plus the portion size eaten to describe just how high and how fast blood sugar might rise with that food). They may be useful as you try to get a handle on how your child's blood glucose responds to particular foods.

Glycemic load

A way of measuring how much and how fast a given portion of food will raise blood sugar.

115

54. Do I need to eliminate all sugar from my child's diet?

No — and quite frankly, we suggest you don't even consider trying. While sugar doesn't help with diabetes control, it shouldn't be regarded as an enemy to be shunned, particularly because there are times when it can be lifesaving in the event of severe hypoglycemia. But aside from that consideration, attempting to eliminate sugar from your child's existence is a doomed effort. You might be able to control everything your children eat while they're small, but as they grow older and interact with other children at school, at the other kids' houses, and in public, it will become impossible to keep tabs on all of their food intake. *Nor should you want to!* It isn't emotionally healthy for a child to grow up with a mother or father who hovers over every bite.

Sugar is everywhere in our culture, and attempting to banish it from your child's life will only backfire; sooner or later, your child will encounter sweets and find that he or she really likes them, and then it becomes a cat-and-mouse game of the child hiding the treats from the parent and the parent trying to second-guess the child's behavior. This is both physically and emotionally unhealthy for all concerned, as it probably will lead to higher (and possibly uncorrected) blood sugars, stress for both parents and child, and a relationship founded on dishonesty and lack of respect.

What you *can* do is keep sugar in its proper place: as an *occasional* (not daily) treat given in small amounts. Whenever possible, foods high in sugar should be paired with a protein — nuts, milk, cheese, or meat. Ideally, your child would only eat a treat after having had a meal, so that there would be less temptation or opportunity to overindulge. But you need to be aware that this rule of thumb must extend to the whole family, not just the child with diabetes, because if your child sees that everyone else gets to have sugar at will when he or she cannot, it will simply cause resentment, frustration, anger... and possibly motivate "sneaking" of sugar, with all the drawbacks we mentioned earlier.

If you want to offer sweets that don't have quite the same glucose "kick" to them, there are plenty of "low carb" offerings that are made with artificial sweeteners such as sucralose, which does not increase blood glucose substantially. If artificial sweeteners concern you or give your child an upset stomach, look into foods made with xylitol, agave nectar, coconut crystals, or stevia leaf (all natural sweeteners with a limited glycemic index).

55. Are there other foods my child shouldn't eat?

In general, your child can eat anything you offer—although *can* isn't the same as *should*. Ideally, you want to promote a healthy mix of foods, with emphasis on fruits, vegetables, nuts, and lean meats, especially fish. If you can see fit to limit some of the common high-sugar or high-carb foods Americans typically eat to occasional (or better yet, rare) use, it will benefit your child—and by that of course we mean soda, candy, ice cream, cake, chips, french fries, and junk food in general, but also white bread, breakfast cereal (especially sugary varieties), pizza, mashed potatoes, and other high-carbohydrate foods you might not necessarily consider "junk", but which are loaded with simple carbs. A great rule of thumb is to avoid anything that includes white flour, sugar, or high fructose corn syrup as one of the first five ingredients, and steer instead toward whole grains and sugar-free foods.

Celiac disease

An autoimmune response in the gut triggered by a protein found in wheat, rye, and barley. People with Type 1 diabetes have an increased risk of developing celiac disease.

Gluten

A protein found in grains such as wheat, rye, and barley that can trigger an auto-immune response in the digestive tract called celiac disease.

Co-occur

A disease that occurs in tandem with or at the same time as another disease.

If your child develops celiac disease, he or she must completely avoid gluten.

It's important that parents know, however, that some children with diabetes are also diagnosed with a second condition called **celiac disease**, which is an autoimmune response triggered by a protein in wheat, rye, and barley called **gluten**. Celiac **co-occurs** with Type 1 diabetes at a rate of about 12.3%, or roughly 1 in 8, although many children do not have celiac when they're first diagnosed with diabetes (on average, those who develop it do so about 3 to 5 years after their diabetes diagnosis). Although we'll discuss celiac disease in greater depth in Question 95, the main thing you need to know about it when it comes to food is this: If your child has or develops celiac disease, he or she must completely avoid products made with wheat, barley, rye, or other forms of gluten. Essentially, that means no breads, cakes, cookies, cereals, noodles, or pastas unless they are made from 100% corn or rice, or using alternative flours such as amaranth or buckwheat (which, despite the misleading name, is a berry rather than a grain). Oats and oatmeal are another possibility as long as you're careful about shopping for steel-cut, organic, certified gluten-free oats—anything else is probably processed in a plant that also processes grains that contain gluten, and even slight cross-contamination can trigger an immune response.

Going gluten-free isn't easy, but it can be and has been done successfully by thousands of people with celiac disease. We list resources for gluten-free living in our Appendix.

56. How do I determine the carbohydrate count of different foods?

There are three factors in calculating carbohydrate counts when your child sits down to eat something: first, how many carbohydrates are there in a serving of the food;

second, how much of the food constitutes a single serving; and third, how many servings is your child going to eat?

Packaging on store-bought foods makes determining the carbohydrate content simple. You simply look at the nutrition facts label (see **Figure 5**) and spot the carbohydrates-per-serving entry, then look at the serving size segment of the label to determine what constitutes a serving. Be aware that for some foods, multiple servings are represented in a package that your child might eat in one sitting—a bag of potato chips, for example, could represent more than one serving, as shown on the label in Figure 5. So if your child eats the whole bag, which is usually the case, you'll need to multiply the number of servings by the carb count per serving to get the child's total carbohydrate intake.

Nutrition Facts

Serving Size 1 ounce   Servings in bag 4

Amount Per Serving

Calories 155   Calories from Fat 93

	% Daily Value*
Total Fat 11g	16%
Saturated Fat 3g	15%
Trans Fat	
Cholesterol 0mg	0%
Sodium 148mg	6%
Total Carbohydrate 14g	5%
Dietary Fiber 1g	5%
Sugars 1g	
Protein 2g	
Vitamin A 0% • Vitamin C	9%
Calcium 1% • Iron	3%

* Percent Daily Values are based on a 2,000 calorie diet. Your daily values may be higher or lower depending on your calorie needs.

Figure 5
Nutrition facts label.

Some foods, like juice, yogurt, cereal, peanut butter, and so forth, will have serving sizes in cups or tablespoons that you'll need to measure out. This is best done with pre-marked measuring cups or spoons (although, over time, you'll probably learn to accurately "eyeball" a full cup or tablespoon of food or liquid). Get to know the standard conversions from cups to ounces (liquid) and from ounces to grams (weight) — it can make life a lot easier if you know that your child's 16-ounce glass of milk at the restaurant translates to 2 cups when the carb-counter book you use gives serving sizes in cups, not ounces.

Home-cooked foods, restaurant foods, or naturally occurring foods like fruits, vegetables, present a little bit of a problem, as recipes and menus generally don't include carbohydrate content or serving size (and every apple or pear is different), but there are resources to help you estimate the carb count. Books such as the Calorie King guide provide the calorie, carbohydrate, and fat content of many foods, fresh as well as prepared, and include standard restaurant menu items for popular chains. There are also many carbohydrate counter tools available in bookstores and online (see the Appendix). These references are often aimed at people trying to follow a low-carb program such as the Atkins diet, but they work just as well for people managing diabetes. In these instances, you are given the carbs per serving by the book or web page, but you'll have to estimate how many servings are in the portion of food you cooked or ordered. A good way of measuring the size of a portion of food is based on your hand: your thumb from the first knuckle to the fingertip represents about 1 ounce of food, the palm of your hand (if you're an average-size woman) is about 3 ounces—for an average-size man, make that 4 ounces—and your closed fist represents about 1 cup. At restaurants, you can either ask the server to measure out 1 cup of your child's beverage or ask them to put it into a cup of known size (8 oz, 10 oz, 12 oz, etc.) so you can estimate how much there is.

Over time, you'll get a sense of what the average carb count of many popular foods should be. A cup (8 oz) of milk usually has about 12 g of carbohydrate, a slice of wheat or whole-grain bread has 20–23 g, a slice of American cheese has 1–2 g, and a handful of potato chips has perhaps 10 g. Though it may be a little tedious at first, over time you'll find that you are automatically totaling up the carb counts in your head without even realizing you're doing it!

Of course, you can't be expected to know the carb content of *everything*, and there will be times when your child has a meal for which you have no idea what the carb content could be. If you have to "guesstimate" the carb count, it's not the end of the world—just be aware that you might be over- or under-estimating the carb content and be ready to treat a low or a high. In these instances, it's helpful to check the child's blood sugar about an hour after the meal to see where it is in relation to where it started out. If it's higher than the original blood sugar, wait another hour or 2 and check again so you can correct if necessary. If it's the same or lower, then you probably gave too much insulin and should ask the child to drink a few ounces of juice, and check again in a couple of hours to be sure the blood sugar level hasn't gone too far in the other direction.

57. How many carbs should my child eat at each meal? How do I make sure he gets the right amount?

Carbohydrates are a necessary part of good nutrition, and your child needs them, but at the same time there's such a thing as too many carbohydrates in the diet (especially when carbs are eaten in place of protein, fiber, and fats).

A healthy adult who eats 2,000 calories a day and does not need to restrict carbohydrates for weight loss generally eats about 180–230 g of carbohydrate daily—a little less than half of the total caloric intake, in other words. For a child, who generally needs a lot less food than an adult until the teen years, it's best as a general rule to make carbohydrates about 50% of the food you provide, with the rest being protein, fiber, and fats. Keep in mind, however, what we mentioned in Question 23: Not all carbohydrates are the same, and complex carbohydrates are better for your child in the long run than simple carbs. If you can manage to make 75% or more of the carbs your child takes in complex carbs rather than simple carbs (not including anything given to treat hypoglycemia!), you're doing pretty well.

The best way to make sure your child gets the right amount of the right *kind* of carbs is to follow the general nutritional guidelines of the USDA. Offer whole grains, fruits, vegetables, lean meats, nuts, eggs, and dairy, and limit sweets and junk food as best you can (especially avoid soda and candy except when treating lows). To that we'd also add, avoid pre-packaged snack foods and frozen dinners, as they frequently use a lot of sugar and are higher in simple carbs than they might appear.

58. What do I do if my child refuses to eat or eats too much?

Eating "too much" is a matter of perception—the parent's perception. Remember that your child is growing and may actually *require* what you consider to be an excessive amount of food to support the energy needs of a developing body. Assuming your child is of normal weight and body mass index (BMI), as long as the child gets sufficient insulin to cover the carbs in the meal, and is getting sufficient exercise to maintain insulin sensitivity (see Question 60), whatever your child eats to satisfy his or her hunger is the right amount, even if *you* think it's too much. If your child is in the habit of overeating out of boredom or other emotional causes, that's a mental health concern that you need to address, but again, it's not a *diabetes* concern as long as the child gets sufficient insulin and stays fit. As we noted in Question 51, a well-balanced diet is always important, but the absolute *amount* of food the child consumes isn't a major issue if he or she is at least eating regular meals.

Of greater concern is a situation in which a child with diabetes skips meals or refuses to eat. This is often an issue with teenagers, for whom "breakfast" may be a dirty word, but young children can be picky and arbitrary about what and when they'll eat too. Food is one of those places that turn into a battleground for many parents, simply because parents and children have very different ideas as to what constitutes "good" food. But whatever else you do, it's important that you *do not let food become a source of conflict between you and your child*. If you get into a power struggle with your child over food, you'll lose. Children figure out pretty quickly that parents won't use the old trick of saying "This is your dinner; eat it or go hungry" when diabetes is involved, because while a child without diabetes might not be harmed by missing a meal, a child with diabetes could have a serious low as a result.

With young children, refusing to eat is often a way of expressing control over their situation. They simply do not understand that refusing food can hurt them. The secret to getting them to eat usually is to offer a wide variety of foods and let them eat what they wish without making a big fuss about it—it's a way of allowing them to feel that they are in charge of what and when they eat.

Older children are capable of understanding the consequences of not eating, and may be more amenable to keeping a regular eating routine as a result. But even the most conscientious teen responds better to your insistence that they have breakfast if you make a point of keeping different foods available for them to choose from—particularly foods that they can "eat on the run." This may force you to compromise somewhat on the nutritional value of the food. If your teen will accept a Pop-Tart for breakfast when he or she might otherwise skip food altogether, then provide Pop-Tarts even if it pains you! But make sure that other options, including bananas, milk, cereal, eggs, bacon, and so on are also available, and continue to encourage your child to take them (even if you know that your encouragement will fall on deaf ears).

As adults, our ideas about what our children should and shouldn't eat are formed by what we were taught by our parents, and by what's considered acceptable in the society around us. You may have had the idea of feeding your child a balanced diet using only the most nutritious foods available, only to have to jettison that idea when your child refuses to eat anything but chicken nuggets. Keep offering your child a variety of foods and, more importantly, make sure *you* eat a varied, healthy diet so you can "model" what good nutrition looks like. *But don't let the child's refusal to eat what you want him or her to eat become a point of contention.* Sooner or later, your picky eater will come around and start eating whatever is offered.

59. What if my child eats food that I haven't covered with insulin?

When your child eats food that for some reason you haven't covered with insulin — either because your child ate it without your knowledge, or because for one reason or another you were unable to offer insulin beforehand or while the child was eating — you have a couple of choices for how to deal with it. If you have a pretty good idea what the child ate and how much insulin it needed, go ahead and deliver the insulin for that food as a single bolus. Your child's blood sugar might go higher than you'd like because of the delay in getting the bolus, but at least the insulin needed to process the glucose will be on its way (better late than never, in this case!). Just remember that your child's blood glucose readings won't fully account for the presence of insulin until at least 2 to 3 hours after the bolus was given, so if you take a reading 1½ hours later, the blood sugar will still be considerably higher than normal—but *do not correct it* because it may eventually come down as a result of the insulin that's still on board.

If you don't know what the child ate or how much insulin the food called for, your best option is to wait about 2 hours, then take a blood sugar reading and correct the high blood glucose reading you'll get at that time. The reason you need to wait that long is that it takes about 2 hours for most of the carbohydrate in the food to enter the bloodstream as glucose (although if the food your child ate also contained a lot of protein or fat, you may need to wait 30 minutes to an hour longer).

60. What is insulin resistance, and how do we avoid it or correct it?

Insulin resistance is a condition in which the body's cells do not respond to insulin as they should. It is the principal issue in Type 2 diabetes, which we discussed briefly in Question 5. Insulin resistance for short periods of time is a normal response to certain hormones—human growth hormone, for example, which is why your child might have a series of high blood sugars while going through a growth spurt—but what we're talking about here is pathological insulin resistance, the sort that signals that Type 2 diabetes is developing.

Long-term, pathological insulin resistance usually develops when two circumstances occur regularly over very long periods of time (usually years or decades): 1) the cells are exposed to high "spikes" of insulin as a result of a diet high in carbohydrates, particularly simple (fast-acting) carbohydrates, and 2) there is insufficient demand by the cells for the high levels of glucose present from the high-carb diet, so most of it gets stored as fat.

Under these conditions, the cells start to ignore the activity of insulin when it tries to introduce glucose into the cells. It's the same reaction you might have if a persistent, annoying neighbor keeps coming to your house to convince you that you should sign a petition you're just not interested in—after a while, you start to dodge him, avoid his phone calls, and refuse to come to the door when he knocks. If he's particularly persistent you'll eventually (reluctantly) let him talk to you in the doorway, but you might not let him all the way into your house.

In a similar fashion, when cells are repeatedly exposed to high levels of insulin, after a while they start to become slow to respond or even stop responding altogether. If they don't respond, eventually they starve; if they respond slowly, some of the glucose that had been waiting around to provide energy gets stored as fat instead. As a result, an insulin-resistant person tends to gain weight and feel mildly fatigued, setting up a self-sustaining cycle of too little exercise and increasing insulin resistance unless they take steps to reverse the cycle through exercise and dietary changes.

To a certain extent, a propensity for insulin resistance is genetic—that is, children who have insulin resistance or Type 2 diabetes in their family health history are considerably more likely to be at risk of developing insulin resistance than those who don't. But since Type 2 diabetes frequently occurs in people with no family history, you can't count on a diabetes-free ancestry to protect your child from developing this complication. So it's better to take steps to limit the risks posed by a high carb diet and limited exercise, whether you have a family history of insulin resistance or not.

Of course, making sure that your child eats a balanced diet and gets sufficient exercise may be easier said than done in many cases, but even if your child is a vegetable-hater, don't despair. Simply make an effort to balance carbohydrates in each meal with a little bit of protein (and fiber, if you can manage it) to help limit the blood sugar "spike" by slowing down the absorption of the food. So if your child wants some cookies, make them conditional upon drinking a glass of milk with them (and, if possible, offer a lower glycemic cookie like oatmeal raisin instead of, say, chocolate chip); if French fries are on the menu, insist that a burger or hot dog be eaten along with them. Save white bread for "special occasions" and make your day-to-day sandwich loaf a whole-wheat or whole-grain brand—and the higher its protein and fiber content, the better.

As far as exercise is concerned, keeping your child active enough to avoid insulin resistance may require you to set some ground rules about television, video game and computer usage, to name three of the prime suspects in the decline of activity among children. But just like the rest of us, children won't exercise if they don't enjoy it, so you'll need to encourage your child to do whatever activity he or she considers fun. It may mean signing your child up for swimming or tennis lessons, or it could be something as simple as turning your living room (and your stereo) over to your adolescent daughter for "dance hour" three nights a week... and yes, it might mean gritting your teeth and tolerating music you consider horrible!

If your child isn't naturally inclined toward athletic pursuits, you may have to get creative in encouraging him or her to exercise—but remember that it doesn't have to be 2 hours of high-intensity sports every day. A simple 30-minute walk or bike ride three or four times a week is sufficient to keep most children fit if they're eating a reasonably balanced diet (and if yours isn't, then you may need some help from a nutritionist as well). For a child who is quiet or scholarly, walking to and from the library or bookstore with you might be all the incentive required.

Should your child develop insulin resistance, exercise and dietary management become that much more important. Unless insulin resistance becomes entrenched, it can usually be reversed through balancing the diet and getting regular exercise. In extreme cases, though, management with drugs that increase insulin sensitivity (for example, Metformin) may be called for.

PART FOUR

Sick Days

How does illness affect my
child's blood sugar?

Should I change my child's insulin
dose during an illness?

Why is vomiting considered a medical
emergency in a child with diabetes?

More . . .

61. How does illness affect my child's blood sugar?

In very simple terms, when your child is sick, extra energy is required to help the immune system fight off an infection. If that were the only factor, parents could simply increase the amount of food and insulin the child takes in, and that would be that…but unfortunately it isn't. For one thing, every child's reaction to illness is different, and might even be different from illness to illness in the same child, so you have to carefully watch trends in your child's blood sugar readings to discover whether the child is trending low or high because of the infection. If you're lucky, your child will be consistent in having either low or high blood sugar readings every time he or she is getting sick, but it's not at all unusual for a child to catch one bug and develop low blood sugar readings while sick, then a few months later catch another one and be through the roof much of the time! So it may take you some time to learn what your child's sick-day patterns are—if there are any patterns to be found.

Sick children often have less interest in food, and the decreased carb intake may also mean lower blood sugar—which can be a major concern if your child is already having low blood sugar readings because of the infection, and a lesser concern (though still a concern) if your child's blood glucose is consistently high. The important consideration here is whether the child is taking in enough food (and insulin) to get sufficient energy to prevent the body from turning to fat-burning for the energy it needs to fight the infection.

What this means for you as a parent is that you need to be watchful. Take your child's blood glucose a little more

REMEMBER

When a child who is on a pump has ketones, you should not deliver an insulin bolus via the pump—use a syringe instead. Reason: Ketones are a sign that insulin delivery is impaired. Check for bubbles in the tubing and change the pump site before you resume using the pump.

frequently, particularly if the child has little appetite. Be sure to monitor ketones every 6–8 hours or so as well, or more often if you're dealing with a combination of poor appetite and lower blood glucose readings—and don't let "normal" blood glucose readings give you a false sense of security, because ketoacidosis can still occur in a sick child whose blood sugar numbers are within the normal range.

One helpful technique is to offer your child plenty of fluids, preferably easy-to-digest drinks with simple carbs in them so that you can keep both blood glucose and insulin moving into the child's system. This serves two purposes: It makes sure enough carbs are coming into the bloodstream to provide energy for the immune system's fight, and it also keeps the child from becoming dehydrated—and if the child has a respiratory infection, the fluids also help thin mucus so the child can breathe better. Gingerale, apple or pear juice, Gatorade, and similar drinks are all good choices; if possible, avoid anything with milk in it because it's harder to digest, and stay away from anything with caffeine because it prevents the child from resting (although if the child won't take anything else, then go ahead and offer these too). In winter, warm beverages like peppermint or ginger tea sweetened with sugar or honey are a good option for either respiratory or stomach bugs because they are soothing to both the head *and* stomach.

The important thing is to ensure that your child's immune system can get the energy it needs without burning fat.

If a sore throat makes it uncomfortable for the child to swallow, turn to popsicles—or, in a pinch, measure some juice or gingerale into your ice cube tray, freeze it, and let your child suck on the ice cubes (you can figure out how many carbs per cube by dividing the number of cubes in a tray by the amount of carbs in the juice you measured out). Or, make a "slush" by putting the frozen juice through a blender. The important thing is that you continue to get both carbohydrates and insulin into your child while he or she is sick—that's the best way to ensure that your child's immune system has the energy it needs without burning fat to get it.

62. Should I change my child's insulin dose during an illness?

Whether your child's insulin dose needs to change during an illness depends on what sort of patterns you're seeing, and if you're the parent of a newly diagnosed child, this is the kind of change that needs to be made in concert with your diabetes team. In other words, *call your team before you start altering the dosages.*

That said, as many experienced parents will tell you, it's pretty common to change insulin dosing when a child is clearly sick. If the child is consistently high for a couple of days when it's obvious from the symptoms that he or she has developed a nasty cold, there's no reason not to make judicious increases to either the basal insulin, the bolus insulin, or both, if only to make the child feel better (a stuffy head is bad enough without having to deal with a hyperglycemic headache on top of it).

For example, a boy who gets his basal insulin by a dose of 3 units of long-acting insulin every 24 hours might do well on 3.5 units when blood sugar is consistently high, with or without changes to the bolus amounts. Or, if this proves too little improvement, carb ratios might be changed so he gets more insulin for the food he eats—so for instance, if this boy gets 1 unit of rapid-acting insulin for every 15 grams of carbohydrate he eats, his parents might change the ratio to 1 unit: 12 grams for the duration of the illness so that he's getting more insulin overall to help bring his blood glucose levels down. In both cases, they would likely change back to the original ratios and doses when lower blood sugars and/or decrease in symptoms show the illness to be past.

Alternatively, let's say a girl who is a pump-user normally has her basal rate set at 0.2 units per hour and a carb ratio of 1 unit: 20 carbs. If she's trending low, her parents could do one of two things: increase her carb ratios, perhaps to 1: 30, so she gets less insulin for the food she eats, or set a lower temporary basal rate of perhaps 0.15 for 3 or 4 hours and see if that brings her blood sugar levels up—or they could try both strategies at the same time. In either case, her parents would want to try to coax her to drink juice or gingerale so they can give her insulin, and they'd be extra cautious about monitoring her ketones and keeping tabs on her blood sugar.

63. Why is vomiting considered a medical emergency in a child with diabetes?

Vomiting is often described as a "medical emergency" in a child with diabetes because of how it affects blood sugar. Sickness often causes blood sugar to drop because the body needs more energy to fight off the illness, but when vomiting occurs, it means that there is no source of additional glucose coming into the system to bring the blood sugar back up—so hypoglycemia is a very strong possibility. Moreover, if nausea prevents the child from eating or drinking anything containing carbs, there is no opportunity to give insulin, so the body turns to fat-burning for fuel, resulting in elevated ketones. Dehydration is also a possibility if your child can't keep fluids down, and dehydration reduces the cells' response to insulin—which increases the likelihood of ketoacidosis.

If your child vomits once but recovers quickly and continues to have an appetite, don't panic. Offer the child stomach-friendly foods that contain plenty of carbohydrates: gingerale, Gatorade, or low-acid juice (apple or pear, not orange juice or lemonade), and if the child feels able to eat solid foods, plain toast, rice, or bananas (all of which are easy on the stomach and high in carbs). If the child feels even a little bit nauseous, consider giving only half the insulin dose the food would require and wait to give the other half till the child has been 30 minutes to an hour without throwing up. The goal is to get food in and keep it in so that you can continue to give enough insulin to keep ketones away, but not so much that you bring on a low. You might also consider lowering the bolus amount (or the basal rate, if the child is on a pump). And make sure you know where your glucagon shot is, just in case!

Elizabeth's comment:

All children are susceptible to viruses that make them vomit, so understand that this is something you'll eventually have to deal with. It sounds pretty scary at first, but you start to understand what you need to do after the first couple of times you deal with vomit-bugs. But sick days with vomiting will be INFINITELY easier if you prepare for them ahead of time. Here are some tips: First, make sure that you always keep a glucagon kit in the house (and make a point of checking the expiration date regularly so you can refill it before it expires). Glucagon was my saving grace the first time Eric had a really serious stomach virus. Second, keep a store of gingerale, juice, or Gatorade, preferably in small-serving cans or pouches, that is designated as the "emergency stash" that is not to be used for any reason except illness (so you have it handy for those times your child suddenly gets sick in the middle of the night when you're not able to run out and get some!). Also, check with your doctor on whether it's appropriate to prescribe an anti-emetic like Zofran®—for small children, it's available as a liquid rather than tablets, and even though we don't like using it because it's pretty powerful stuff, it's saved us a couple of times when Eric otherwise would've been in serious trouble from stomach viruses or flu. I was very grateful to have it when Eric came down with swine flu in the fall of 2009! And beyond that, just make sure you keep a close eye on blood sugar and ketones till the sickness passes.

64. How often should I test blood sugar and ketone levels when my child becomes ill?

Illness doesn't automatically mean more testing; for the most part, you should continue your usual testing routine unless you start to see signs that the illness is starting to affect your child's blood sugar levels. For example, if you normally test at mealtimes but find that your child experiences low blood sugars an hour or so before you'd normally test, it may become necessary to test more often so you can give your child some carbs when you catch a low coming on. This would also be a good time to do a ketone check even if your routine doesn't normally call for one.

Testing blood glucose every 1 to 2 hours, or even more often, is not unusual in a sick child, particularly when the illness causes the child to feel nauseous or refuse food. Such frequent testing may be uncomfortable for the child, but it's one key to avoiding blood sugar crashes or DKA. If you test frequently and find no abnormal results, however, it's OK to cut back to make your child

When your child is sick, be sure to check ketones at least every 6-8 hours.

more comfortable. Also, be sure to check ketones at least every 6–8 hours when a child is sick. If there are ketones, contact your diabetes center for advice on how to address the problem. You should probably plan on checking for ketones again 2 to 2½ hours after you treat for ketones to assess whether any further action is necessary.

65. Can my child take over-the-counter medications? What about prescription drugs?

Many medications, whether prescription or over-the-counter, are as safe for children with diabetes as they are for children without diabetes. However, there are a number of medications that can affect blood sugar. Decongestants that include pseudoephedrine, for example, can raise blood sugar; so can corticosteroids, which are sometimes used in asthma treatment. Some steroid medications, such as prednisolone, not only raise blood sugar but temporarily cause insulin resistance, so that the child's insulin use increases substantially while this medication is being used. ADHD medications in the methylphenidate family (Ritalin and Concerta, to name two) can cause a marked drop in blood glucose levels after administration. So before you give your child certain medications, it's a good idea to check with either your pharmacist or your endocrinologist on whether the ingredients in the medication will alter blood sugar. This doesn't mean you cannot use them if there aren't any better alternatives, but it may mean that you have to be careful about checking blood sugar and offering either food or insulin as appropriate to counteract any effects it might have after it's given.

66. If my child is ill or injured, should I call the pediatrician or the endocrinologist first?

The usual childhood illnesses don't require an intervention by the endocrinologist, so the first person to call is your child's pediatrician. The exception to this rule of thumb comes when the illness has a strong impact on the child's blood sugar levels and ketones, as described in Questions 63 and 64. Any time your child has a virus that causes low blood sugars, or high blood sugars with ketones, it's a good idea to check in with your diabetes team to let them know what's happening and get their advice for next steps. But even in these situations, the pediatrician may still be your first stop.

Unusual illnesses—whether they be infectious diseases like meningitis, acute conditions like appendicitis, or a long-term illness like cancer—will also be treated first by your pediatrician, and then (if necessary) by a specialist, but the presence of the additional health problem should be brought to the attention of your endocrinologist as soon as possible so that he or she can work with your pediatrician or specialist to treat the disease while monitoring your child's blood sugar levels.

Keep in mind that most pediatricians do not know everything about Type 1 diabetes. If you get advice from the pediatrician that you feel might cause problems with managing your child's blood sugar, play it safe and get a second opinion from the endocrinologist.

Injuries ranging from cuts and scrapes to sprains and fractures are also something for your pediatrician to look after, unless they're severe enough to warrant a trip to the emergency room (and even then, you should notify your pediatrician en route to the hospital). Although the stress of a severe injury like a broken bone usually raises your child's blood sugar, it may also drop your child's blood sugar rapidly as the immune system calls for more energy to deal with the injury. So it's crucial to make sure that the emergency responders (and later, the ER physicians) know to check the child's blood sugar and provide juice, a glucose drip, or insulin to keep blood glucose levels stable while the child is in their care. If the injury is extremely severe (a head injury or multiple broken bones from a car crash, for instance), get word to your child's pediatrician *and* endocrinologist so that both can advise the first responders and the ER team on the best way to treat the injury while keeping your child's blood sugar stable.

Once the injury is stabilized, your next priority is checking blood glucose levels and making sure that blood glucose stays in range en route. If your child is conscious, this just means making sure he or she continues to eat and drink carbs as necessary, and giving small amounts of insulin to offset the carbs (otherwise the energy won't get to the cells that need it). If your child isn't conscious, the emergency rescue team can put the child on an intravenous glucose drip, which you will then need to counteract with small corrective doses of insulin. Have the paramedic or ER physician help you to calculate the dose, since they will know better than you how much glucose is going into your child's body during the time it takes from the start of the drip to your arrival at the hospital. If that's not possible, you can use cake gel inside the gums to keep blood sugar stable, or turn to your glucagon shot if blood glucose falls below the minimum safe level en route to the hospital.

After you get to the hospital, continue to make it clear to anyone and everyone who comes anywhere near your child that he or she has diabetes—otherwise, you can't be certain that the word gets passed from one team to the next that monitoring blood glucose is necessary. If the injury is bad enough to require surgery, insist that they consult either your endocrinologist or, failing that, an endocrinologist knowledgeable about Type 1 diabetes—they'll need this type of expertise to manage your child's blood sugars during and after surgery.

Be aware that healing from an injury or surgery tends to be slower in people with diabetes than in people without diabetes, and the possibility of infection is a very serious consideration. You and your child need to be very diligent about following the medical team's recommendations for recovery, particularly when it comes to broken bones or open wounds. You may also find that the diabetes regimen you used prior to the injury changes somewhat, because your child will need more energy and more insulin while the healing process is underway. That's something you should discuss with your endocrinologist.

Elizabeth's comment:

I've never been one of those parents who drags their kid off to the doctor at the slightest sniffle, but Eric's diabetes has made me a lot quicker to call the pediatrician than I used to be, particularly when it comes to infections. One thing I particularly want parents to know is how important it is to take care of cuts and other wounds quickly. You don't have to do anything fancy, just soap and water and a Band-aid, or some antibiotic ointment if it's particularly deep—but it IS important that you take care of it and keep it clean, because the danger of infection is a lot higher than you might think.

And don't be afraid to take your child to the doctor for an infected cut, because you'd be amazed at how fast an infection can go systemic. The first sign of redness and swelling in a pump site, a bug bite, or a cut isn't generally enough to warrant a visit, but if I get aggressive with the antibiotic ointment and it still doesn't go away or go down within a day, that's when I take Eric in to see his doctor. Eric has had a pump site get infected and lead to a systemic infection before, and it's not an experience I want to repeat—and my pediatrician agrees with me that when it comes to infections, it's better to bring him in for something that turns out to be minor than to keep him home and find out the hard way that I should have brought him in.

PART FIVE

Daily Life with Diabetes

Will my child ever be able to do all
the things other kids can do?

Will my child be able to participate
in sports and other activities?

Does my child need to wear a medical ID
bracelet or necklace?

More . . .

67. Will my child ever be able to do all the things other kids can do?

Your child can do everything any child without diabetes can do.

Absolutely! Your child can do everything any child without diabetes can do. The main difference is that your child needs to be more conscientious about what and when he or she eats, and be mindful of how the day's activities affect insulin needs and blood sugar.

Children with diabetes go to daycare, public school, and universities; they participate in sports (see Question 68); they play, go to friends' houses, date, shop, and learn to drive. To do these things, they need to take extra precautions and always need to have insulin, a blood glucose meter, and a carb source available ... all of which can easily be carried in a purse or backpack. They occasionally need cooperation from school officials or activities directors, which might mean a little educating on your part. Beyond that, however, there's no reason at all that children with diabetes shouldn't be able to do anything they wish.

Diabetes is a disease your child has, not a word that describes who he or she is.

As you read this book, one phrase you'll never see is "diabetic child"—it's always "child with diabetes." The reason for that is simple: Diabetes is a disease your child has, not a word that describes who he or she is. Although there will be times when it seems your whole life revolves around it, *diabetes is not the center of your child's life, and it shouldn't be MADE the center of your child's life.* More importantly, it should not be seen as an obstacle to the things your child wants to do with his or her life—not by you, and not by your child. There is nothing more tragic than neglecting a child's goals, talents, or dreams simply because of a disease like diabetes, and we urge parents to do your best to ensure your child is never a "diabetic child" in your mind, your child's mind, or the minds of the people in your child's daily life.

Elizabeth's comment:

Our first day in the pediatric ward, I overheard a nurse refer to Eric as "the diabetic" while she and the other nurses were discussing who would look after which patients that morning. I felt like someone had stuck a knife in me—I didn't want my little son to be "the diabetic" all his life. It seemed so restrictive to pigeonhole him like that when "diabetic" didn't come close to describing his dynamic personality, even at 18 months old!

It wasn't long after that I found the online support group I use, Tudiabetes.org, and realized that people with Type 1 diabetes can live the same full, rich lives other people live if they simply decide that that's what they want to do. So now my husband and I make a point of integrating diabetes into Eric's life—not the other way around. We are determined that Eric is going to participate in any activity he wishes and, if we have anything to say about it, he will never be excluded because of his diabetes. Of course, we'll have no control over what the other kids do or say to him as he grows up and goes to school, but we can at least make sure he understands that their prejudices don't reflect anything about his worth—and that he has our love and support at all times.

68. Will my child be able to participate in sports and other activities?

Your child is able to participate in sports and activities, but you will need to make sure that the coaches or coordinators of the activity are aware that your child has diabetes and understand what that means. A preseason meeting with the staff is probably the best place to explain these facts—we certainly recommend you don't wait until the first practice, because a coach with 10 or 15 eager kids to direct isn't going to be in the mood to sit and listen to you describe the ins and outs of diabetes care!

If you can arrange such a meeting, this is a good time to tell the coaching staff a few of the realities of Type 1 diabetes. The coach needs to know, for instance, that your child may require food or sports drinks during the course of games or practices to keep blood sugar levels from crashing—keep in mind that strenuous exercise will tend to lower blood sugar. The coach will also need to understand that your child's blood sugars will need to be checked periodically—by you, if the child isn't already handling his or her own care, but for older kids (high school age, in general), this can also be handled by the coaching staff with very little training. More than anything, however, the coaching staff needs to be aware that your child's diabetes *doesn't affect his or her athletic ability*. There are plenty of athletes with Type 1 diabetes playing in all levels of sports, including professional baseball and football and several Olympic-caliber athletes.

Coaches may be reluctant or even fearful of letting your child play, but if you are patient and help them to recognize that your child's medical situation needs only a few relatively minor adjustments to ensure safety, you should be able to convince them that it will be okay. Bear in mind that the more confident *you* are about this, the more likely they will be to accept that you know what you're talking about!

Understand that you may need to do a few things differently when your child begins sports. Some of the do's and don'ts of pre-competition blood sugar management include:

Do:

- check your child's blood sugar *and ketones* before the game, and recheck blood sugar at regular intervals during competition

- strive for a slightly higher blood sugar level at game time than you normally would—perhaps 20 to 50 points higher than the upper level of the normal range—so there's less danger of going low during strenuous exercise

- have both water *and* Gatorade or other drinks containing sugars available so that your child can stay hydrated without loading up on carbs *unless they're needed*—in other words, offer only water unless your child's blood glucose makes it clear that more energy is called for

- forbid your child to participate if ketones are present— exercise will make ketones worse and could trigger ketoacidosis

- record blood sugars, carbohydrate intake, and playing time in a log book while your child plays, so you can start to see how patterns of insulin use and carbohydrate needs develop in relation to exercise (which will make future activities easier)

Don't:

- avoid the issue by denying your child permission to be involved in sports

- give your child extra carbs in anticipation of strenuous exercise if you're not certain of the playing time to be distributed by the coach

- allow your child to enter a game or sports activity if blood sugars are low—this could trigger a crash. If the child's blood sugar is in the lower third of his or her range when play starts, give 10 to 15 carbs as a "booster" before he or she takes part

- leave game-day diabetes management in the hands of a coach, coaching staff, or your child unless all of the above are very experienced in how and when to check blood sugar—let them focus on the game, while you keep tabs on blood glucose levels during play

- forget to watch the game and talk to your child about his or her performance afterward—if you are strictly there as the "diabetes police," it can make your child less enthusiastic about competing and decrease the child's overall morale

Sports injuries

Blood sugar is not the only concern when a child with diabetes plays sports; there's also the ever-present possibility of injuries, minor or major. When an injury occurs, the body immediately responds in two ways: first, there is an increase in insulin resistance, and second, glycogen is released from the liver to raise blood glucose. Both of these responses mean that blood glucose levels will rise. That means that most immediate concern if your child is injured or wounded (other than stopping any bleeding, if it's a wound) is preventing hyperglycemia.

Some tips about how to handle injuries:

Minor injuries like a sprained ankle or a small cut probably won't cause significant blood sugar fluctuations unless the child was trending high or low to begin with. Test the child's blood sugar. If your child is in the lower end of the target range, provide a small snack or juice to bring blood sugar up to the middle of the range to avoid any problems with hypoglycemia. If high, correct it with insulin, and check again about an hour later to make sure blood sugar is starting to come down.

Significant injuries involving broken bones or significant bleeding need quick action to manage both the injury and blood sugar. Blood sugar may rise or drop rapidly, so test frequently, provide insulin if needed, or if the blood sugar is trending low, offer juice or glucose tablets if your child is able to take them, or use glucagon if not. **Make sure that any medical personnel or emergency workers who might be summoned are aware that your child has diabetes.**

Make sure any medical personnel or emergency workers are aware that your child has diabetes.

For more on handling injuries, see Question 66.

69. Does my child need to wear a medical ID bracelet or necklace?

Wearing a medical ID bracelet or necklace is generally a necessity for people with diabetes, and your child is no exception. The reason is quite simple: There may come a time when your child experiences a sudden low blood sugar, convulsions, or coma, or is in an accident and needs emergency care. If you are not there (or aren't able) to tell the emergency services personnel what your child needs, this bracelet can make the difference in how fast your child gets treatment suited to a person with diabetes. So we do recommend that you try to keep some form of identification that specifies your child's medical condition on the child at all times.

Getting your child to comply with this directive might be challenging. Particularly in older school-age children and teens, wearing a medical ID might be a source of rebellion or discomfort—another reminder that your child is "different" from his or her friends. So be prepared to negotiate compromises from time to time. For instance, if your daughter is in school, where teachers and staff are aware of her condition, she doesn't need to wear the ID bracelet, but if she's at the mall with her friends, she does—or she can't go. Or, tell your son that he can attach his ID necklace to his belt loop and shove it in his pocket if he doesn't want to wear it around his neck. Make sure they understand *why* you insist they keep it with them, and be firm but understanding if they object.

70. Will my child eventually learn to handle carb counting, injections, and overall diabetes care?

Parents turn diabetes management over to the child when the child is ready for the responsibility, but stay involved enough to offer support and sometimes a break.

This isn't a question of *will* or *won't*—this is a question of *when* and, to a certain extent, *how well*. All adults with Type 1 diabetes had to take over their own care at some point in their lives, and your child will, too. The most important factor to keep in mind, however, is that there's a fine line between pushing your child too hard to be "in charge" (which tends to lead to poor self-care later on; see Questions 96 and 99) and being a "helicopter parent" who spends all your time hovering over your child because you don't trust the child to do it right. The goal for parents is to eventually turn much of the management over to the child when the child is ready for the responsibility, but to stay involved enough to offer the child support, and sometimes a break.

How soon your child can begin learning to handle his or her diabetes care depends in part on how old the child is at diagnosis. Most children under 5 aren't equipped to do very much because they aren't yet able to read and don't have math skills—they can learn to recognize highs and lows, and some can even use the blood glucose meter, but measuring out and injecting insulin, calculating carbs, and so on is something parents will need to do for a while. Children age 4 or 5 are usually able to recognize when they're hypoglycemic, and should be encouraged to care for themselves by alerting you that they need to be checked when they feel low. This is also a good age to start thinking about sending your child to a diabetes camp or, if one is available nearby, a diabetes play group so that your child can interact with other children who have diabetes.

If your child is old enough to have mastered basic math (7 to 9 years old), then he or she can participate in calculating carbs, and depending on the child's comfort level, learn to inject insulin that has been measured out already (for those using syringes) or program a bolus dose into a pump. In both cases, the parent should still closely supervise the child, both to make sure it's done properly and to give the child a sense of safety and encouragement—the idea is to have the child feel good about caring for him/herself. We strongly advise parents not to push these tasks on the child; if the child is uninterested or unwilling to take part in these tasks, it's a clear signal that he or she simply isn't emotionally ready for the responsibility. Even if the child is willing to participate, this age group is too young to safely measure out insulin for injection or to calculate insulin doses, so most of the management tasks must still be performed by a parent or caregiver.

Children older than 10 should be encouraged to learn about their care (but again, not pushed or forced to do it), and certainly most children 13 or older have the ability to do the calculations and insulin delivery tasks and may be ready to actively participate in diabetes management. But even if the child is eager to take up the reins, there are good reasons for parents to stay involved in diabetes management tasks like checking blood sugar, calculating carbs, and delivering insulin.

First, you want to stay involved so you can be sure the child is performing the tasks correctly. Your goal isn't just to teach the child to do the job, but to do the job *well*, and that means you need to make sure that your child can do the calculations properly every time. Bear in mind that adolescence is a time when tremendous changes take place in your child's brain, so even if you see that your son or daughter is doing the calculations properly one day, that doesn't mean that he or she will do them right *every time*. Forgetfulness, fogginess, distraction and (let's face it) out and out ditziness is a hallmark of the rampaging hormones affecting teens—so it's not really a good time for them to be fully on their own with diabetes care!

A second reason is that diabetes care is about more than just the day-to-day tasks of taking blood sugars and calculating insulin doses. The patterns of highs and lows during a week, month, or season can be as important to maintaining good diabetes control as the daily rhythms, but children are rarely able to determine such patterns on their own. By staying involved in their care even after they take up the essential tasks, you can discover these patterns and help them to account for them.

A third reason is so that the child won't get "burnout" as quickly—something that many people with diabetes encounter after they've mastered what to do and are simply doing it day after day. The reality that you're *always* going to have to check your blood sugar, count your carbs, and give yourself insulin before you can sit down and eat sinks in eventually, and it's no fun, particularly if you're a teenager who'd rather be doing something (anything) else. And unless you're a parent who also happens to have diabetes, you can't really empathize with how it feels for your child to have diabetes. Parents, after all, get to *stop* the day-to-day drill when their children grow up and learn to take care of themselves. Children with diabetes may never get to stop, and once they realize this, they frequently rebel against it (see Question 99).

A parent can stay actively involved in the child's diabetes management in a number of ways: by directly supervising (but not performing) the tasks of using a blood glucose meter, calculating insulin doses, and delivering insulin; by reviewing the log book or meter and pump histories daily with the child; or by simply having a nightly "check-in" time with the child so that you can talk about the day's readings and look for patterns together. Depending on how your child feels about managing his or her own care (some are eager, others are reluctant), you can use some or all of these suggestions, or consult with other parents to find what works for them. However you choose to stay involved, it's important that you *do* stay involved—if for no other reason than to give your son or daughter a break from having to constantly think about it while they're in the midst of trying to grow up!

71. What do I tell my child when other children treat him as though he's different because of his diabetes?

As parents, we all know that children can be pretty hard on anyone who is "different," and diabetes can be a pretty big difference—particularly if your child is the only one in his or her school or daycare with diabetes or any other physical disorder. Your child will need reassurance that other children's negative attitudes aren't a reflection that there's anything "wrong" with your child—instead, it shows that they're ignorant, and may even be afraid of what they don't understand. The cure for fear and ignorance is education. If your child can explain to the other children exactly what it is that's "different" about having diabetes, it might help to reduce your child's difficulty in interacting with other children. Diabetes is nothing to be ashamed of, and indeed by "spreading the word" and teaching a peer group about the disease, your child may be helping more than just him- or herself—but this is a message that you may need to reinforce with your child on a regular basis.

Helping your child to teach other children about diabetes has two very helpful "side effects": one, it reinforces what you're trying to teach your child about his or her own condition; and two, it enables your child to get assistance from his or her peers in keeping an eye out for unexpected lows. It's not at all uncommon for children with diabetes who are experiencing a low to be noticed and assisted by their friends, whether that assistance comes in the form of alerting an adult to the child's condition or simply offering a timely piece of candy or a juice box. So we suggest that you encourage your child to explain diabetes to the peer group as a matter of course. For very young children, there are a number of books that can be read at the daycare or in the classroom (most are appropriate for a first- through fifth-grade level). For older children, it might be helpful to ask your diabetes educator to come in at the beginning of each school year to give a short presentation, if you feel that's necessary or appropriate.

Elizabeth's comment:

I had a lot of trouble writing about this subject, because at this stage I had no idea what to say… a toddler isn't really subject to peer rejection, and all of the kids in his daycare have grown fully accustomed to Eric having shots all the time (and now an insulin pump)—so at this point it's not an issue I've encountered. And yet, sooner or later this is something I'm going to have to figure out, because the way kids are, it will come up somewhere down the line, probably when he starts school. I ended up doing a lot of research, talking to other parents on my online chat group, and buying a couple of books on the subject.

What I learned from it is, very simply, that children need to approach other children with honesty and be very up front with them about the disease—in short, to do some educating of their peers. That means that the child needs to understand his or her disease so he or she can explain it. It's a lot easier for children to be accepting of a child made "different" by diabetes if they understand just what diabetes is—when they know WHY the insulin injections or the pump are necessary, and they understand the reason that your child continually needs food during class or before recess, they become much more accepting of these differences. My husband and I have tried to set an example by explaining Eric's condition anytime we go out in public and get questions (restaurants, particularly), and we've gotten terrific feedback from parents and children alike.

I got great information from a book called "Diabetes Through the Looking Glass," which is about how diabetes looks to children with diabetes. It's sponsored by both the JDRF and Diabetes UK, and while it's written by a British physician for a British audience (so some of the advice doesn't really resonate with a U.S. audience), it has a great deal of input from children with diabetes about their feelings and experiences. I think most parents would do well to read it.

72. Can changes in the weather affect my child's blood glucose levels?

Weather tends to affect blood glucose indirectly, by altering two factors: first, the body's responses change according to whether it needs to conserve heat or cool off; and second, children's behavior tends to change depending on weather (and season).

Several factors interact to change blood glucose. These are:

- **Temperature**. Hot, humid weather tends to lead to lower blood glucose levels because the blood vessels dilate to shed excess heat. This makes insulin absorb faster, so it can lead to either unexpected lows or highs. You might see an unexpected low if, for instance, you're giving a bolus 20–30 minutes before a meal on a hot day. Cold weather, also, can affect blood glucose levels and insulin requirements. In general, most parents see an increase in insulin requirements and higher overall blood glucose levels when the seasons change from warm to cool or cold, but at the same time, spending a lot of time outdoors in cool or cold weather can lead to lows. This seeming contradiction is explained by the fact that cold weather tends to make the body shift into heat-conservation mode (constricted blood vessels, a more sluggish metabolism), but at the same time, being out *in* the cold weather demands additional energy to keep warm—so blood sugar burns down faster.

- **Altitude changes**. If you travel to a higher altitude, expect your child's blood glucose levels to drop as the child's metabolism increases to provide more oxygen. You may find that you need to lower the child's basal insulin by 20-40%, but this effect should only last a few days until the child becomes acclimated.

- **Activity levels**. In general, children tend to be more active in warm weather than in cold weather, and activity levels tend to predict blood sugar and insulin requirements.

All of this is fine in theory, but *your* child's response is going to be unique. You'll need to learn over time how your child's body and behavior change with cold or warm weather. Use these generalities as guidelines, but pay attention to what *really* happens when your child is out in hot, cold, rainy, snowy, humid, or dry weather. And bear in mind that any time your child is exposed to extreme weather conditions, it's a good idea to pay special attention to blood sugar levels and hydration.

73. What effects will my daughter's menstrual cycle have on her diabetes control?

The hormonal shifts that accompany the start of a girl's period can play havoc with her blood sugar levels. Many women with diabetes find that they have a few days of higher blood sugars before they start their periods, and then drop lower once menstruation begins. This may or may not be true of your daughter because growth hormones also affect both insulin use and menstruation. However, if she has been cycling regularly for six months or more, she should be able to chart her blood sugars against her cycle to determine how her blood sugars change over the course of a month. If she does this for at least 3 months, a pattern should emerge that will allow you and your daughter to adjust her basal rate upward or downward as needed.

74. Can my child still attend overnight summer camp?

Unless the camp staff is trained and experienced in how to manage diabetes (and most aren't), it's not advisable to let your child attend a standard summer camp—but that doesn't mean that summer camp is altogether out of the question. There are many summer camps that cater specifically to children with special health needs, and quite a few of these specifically serve children with diabetes. The American Camping Association lists 92 such camps in their "find a camp" search feature if you specify only that your child is "special needs–diabetes;" obviously, whether there's a camp located near you depends on where you live, but there are camps in every region of the United States.

Going to a camp that specifically serves children with diabetes can be enormously rewarding for your child. The most significant benefit he or she will get is to experience something that might not be an everyday occurrence—that there are other children "just like me," and that having diabetes doesn't mean missing out on the fun things other kids do. Your child may also learn how to better manage diabetes from other children who have lived with the disease longer.

The American Diabetes Association's position statement on diabetes camps gives a comprehensive list of what parents should expect when sending their child to a diabetes camp. It's worth reviewing this statement, which is available at http://www.childrenwithdiabetes.com/camps/d_07_103.htm. Or you can visit the ADA's web site and review their section on diabetes camps.

75. How do we handle unexpected changes in our routine?

As the saying goes, "expect the unexpected"—which means, be prepared for the curveballs that will sometimes get thrown at you. Here's an example: a flat tire! Suppose that a flat tire happens on the way home from work, and it means you're going to be late getting dinner. In that case, be ready to bend the rules a little and let your child have a pre-dinner snack to avoid the low that might accompany the delay. Or suppose that flat tire should occur on a back road while you're driving with your child to the supermarket. If you're prepared, you have the fully stocked diabetes kit with you (see Question 16), which means you not only can give your child a snack, you can cover that snack with insulin so that neither lows nor highs need occur while you're fixing the flat (or waiting for roadside assistance). If you're *really* prepared, you have a folder containing your child's daily insulin and carb log with you, so you can have a sense of what the unexpected snack will mean for the child's insulin requirements for the rest of the day.

But you'll also need to cut yourself some slack. No matter how hard you try, "stuff happens" that you can't anticipate, and you may wind up dealing with severe highs or lows on occasion. Keep your cool, do what you need to do in order to bring your child's blood glucose level back into range, head for the ER if you absolutely must ... and don't beat yourself up about it. An occasional blood sugar crisis happens to all people with diabetes, no matter how careful or experienced they may be.

No matter how hard you try, "stuff happens" that you can't anticipate, and you may wind up dealing with severe highs or lows on occasion.

CHILDCARE AND EDUCATION FOR A CHILD WITH DIABETES

76. Can my child still attend daycare, after school programs, and public schools?

Diabetes is considered a disability under specific federal laws that make discrimination against disabled persons illegal. These laws are described in Question 77, but in general, they make it illegal for any school, daycare, or after school program (other than those run by religious organizations) to refuse admission to your child simply because of the child's diabetes. Nevertheless, such refusals do occur, and even where schools or centers accept a child with diabetes, they don't necessarily provide appropriate supervision to make sure that the child's blood glucose is properly managed—a truly alarming prospect for parents, especially parents of a newly diagnosed child.

Whether your child can attend a daycare or after school program *safely* really depends on the willingness of the center's managers and teachers to learn about your child's needs, and your own willingness to be flexible. Some daycare centers may be able to accommodate a child with diabetes as far as testing blood glucose regularly and properly feeding the child is concerned, but depending on state law and insurance coverage, they may require that the parent handle insulin injections. Others, concerned about insurance issues if they take on responsibility for managing the child's disease, may require the parent to supervise *all* aspects of managing blood glucose, which in essence negates much of the value of daycare—a working parent can hardly do his or her job if constantly required to run off to the daycare to keep tabs on blood sugar, insulin, and food! So in practice, though the daycare owners or the managers of after school programs might be obligated to accept your child by law, they can make it difficult, if not impossible, for your child's diabetes to be managed well—forcing you, for your child's well-being, to look elsewhere for childcare.

If your child is to attend a daycare or after school pro-gram, it's best to sit down with the center or program's managers, ideally in concert with your diabetes educator, so that the care providers get an accurate idea of what will be expected of them day to day. Although it may take some negotiation, many care providers will work with parents, particularly if the child has already been attending the facility or program prior to the diagnosis. If they won't, however, you may need to look into obtain-ing home care for your child—something that may be a financial burden unless you can make use of services to support it (see **Part Six: Other Things Parents Worry About** for more).

When it comes to public schools, however, parents have a lot more leverage. Public schools are supported by public taxes and are required under the laws listed above, as well as many state and local laws, to accommodate children with special needs. We talk about that more in Ques-tions 77 and 78.

Elizabeth's comment:

We were fortunate in that Eric's daycare provider at the time of his diagnosis had been caring for Eric for 4 months, and his older brother for over a year, when we discovered his diabetes. She had a few reservations about continuing to care for him after the diagnosis, but was willing to work with us to see if we could come up with a routine that would benefit all concerned. This was despite the fact that other people she knew were cautioning her against accepting him back, telling her that she was opening herself up to a lawsuit if anything should happen to Eric while she was caring for him! But with training from our diabetes team and constant communication between her, her staff, my husband, and me, we eventually worked out a routine where she and her staff recorded Eric's blood sugars and food intake and we used those records to analyze his patterns and give him insulin injections during the day. And once he was put on a pump, we got training for her and her staff on how to program it, and now they give him the insulin themselves, only calling me for questions if they see anything unusual, like an unexpected high or low. At this point, Eric's daycare provider knows almost as much about handling Eric's insulin needs as I do. The only thing she ever calls me for is to change his pump site if he should pull it out, or advise her on how to handle unexpected swings in blood sugar, and that's very rare.

I think to a large extent, if they're willing to work with you, the daycare provider will follow your lead when it comes to diabetes management. If you can give them training from your diabetes educator, a routine to follow, and clear instructions as to what they need to do if there's a problem, most of the time they can handle it. But if they're not willing to at least try, then you need to start looking elsewhere—because no amount of training or discussion is going to change that.

As far as the school district is concerned, we're a few years away from that, but my plan is to start talking to the school's staff after Eric's older brother starts kindergarten in the fall to lay the groundwork for Eric's entry into the school system in 2012. I know there are at least three children with Type 1 diabetes in the district—one's in my teenage stepdaughter's class in high school, and two others are in the elementary school where Eric will start kindergarten next year—so this shouldn't be all that novel to them, but I'm still going to make it clear what's coming, and what I expect from the school, so there won't be any surprises. I've heard horror stories about lack of support from the school systems from parents in other parts of the country, but forewarned is forearmed—I have 2 more years to study up on the disability laws, and that's what I intend to do. Knowledge is power, and to a certain extent you have to grit your teeth and be prepared for a fight even while you're hoping to avoid one.

77. How are the rights of children with diabetes protected under law?

Federal disability laws that protect children with diabetes include the following:

The Rehabilitation Act of 1973 (Section 504)

Section 504 of the Rehabilitation Act requires any school that receives federal funds of any kind to provide children with an identifiable disability or impairment—including diabetes—with a plan intended to make sure that the child is able to safely participate in all school activities *and* get appropriate care for their medical needs. Schools can lose federal funding if they do not comply with this law, and a school cannot require parents to waive liability as a condition of giving medicine. Thus, all public schools must work with parents to create such a plan—although we need to stress the point that *the parents must first request the plan* (see Question 78). If you do not submit a letter each year to your school district requesting a plan, the school is not obligated to provide one—so be sure you do your part before the beginning of the school year.

The Americans with Disabilities Act of 1990

The ADA prohibits all schools and daycare centers, except those run by religious organizations, from discriminating against children with disabilities, including diabetes. Protection under this law is the same as that for Section 504.

Individuals with Disabilities Education Act (IDEA)

IDEA requires the federal government to fund state and local education agencies for the education of students with disabilities, including children with diabetes. The school is then required to develop an Individualized Education Plan (IEP) to accommodate your child's needs. What this means, in effect, is that your school district cannot use the expense of supporting your child's special needs as a reason for refusing your request. As with the 504 Plan, you need to notify the school of the need for an IEP in advance of the school year so they have time to create and implement the plan.

State Regulations

Some states have enacted additional legislation to protect children with disabilities. Contact your state legislature for further information.

78. What is a 504 Plan? How do I get a 504 Plan for my child?

504 Plan

A plan created with school officials that spells out what accommodations the school will make to manage the special needs of a child with a legal disability, such as diabetes.

As mentioned in Question 77, Section 504 of the Rehabilitation Act of 1973 requires public schools that accept federal funding to make accommodations for children with disabilities or special needs. A **504 Plan** is a document that spells out what these accommodations will be—and in your child's case, that includes identifying staff who will be in charge of making sure your child's diabetes is managed (especially important in young children who aren't able to manage it themselves).

The 504 Plan for a child with diabetes must include the following information:

- Blood glucose testing procedures (when, where, and by whom). For younger children, this will likely be done by the school nurse in the nurse's office; the Plan should specify an individual to escort the child to see the nurse at predetermined times, or at times that the child seems to be experiencing (or complains of) hypoglycemia. *A child who complains of, or shows signs of, low blood sugar must not go alone to the nurse's office!*

A child who complains of, or shows signs of, low blood sugar must not go alone to the nurse's office!

- For older children who are able to check their own blood glucose levels, particularly those in high school, testing can be a sticking point — schools may be reluctant to allow testing in the classroom, halls, or bathroom, citing safety concerns, yet it's unrealistic to expect an adolescent to hurry to the nurse's office between classes (more likely, the child would skip the test and run the risk of having a low or high blood sugar during class time). The school has the right to restrict blood glucose testing to locations outside of the classroom, but if you can demonstrate that this procedure will not endanger others (for instance, making sure that test strips, wipes, and other materials that come in contact with your child's blood will be disposed of at home and not at school), your school may allow the child to check in a specified place in the classroom.

- A Diabetes Medical Management Plan (see Question 79) that details medication procedures and dosages (including an "insulin roadmap" that details when and how to administer insulin). This plan will specify whether your child is capable of deciding the amount to be given and, if not, provide an alternative such as calling a parent or using a chart to determine the amount to be given.

- Procedures for treatment of hyper- and hypoglycemia
- Precautions to be taken before physical activity. These precautions are not just for gym teachers but include recess, games or activities in the classroom, or field trips that require a great deal of walking.
- Guidelines for meals, snacks, special treats, and parties
- Contact information for medical assistance (as needed) and parents

As a parent of a child with diabetes, it is extremely important that you request a 504 Plan every year that your child attends a public school, because making this request ensures that the school officials and teachers are involved in your child's care and well-being. And above all, it's essential that this request be made *in writing*. A verbal request isn't enough to ensure you get an appropriate response, and it's also something you can't document should there be a problem in developing and implementing the plan.

School districts have different procedures for how a parent must request a 504 Plan. Some have specific request forms to be filled out; others need a letter from the parent detailing the child's disability and asking for a meeting with school officials; still others require a doctor's letter specifying that the child has a particular disability that requires accommodations. It's a good idea to call the school your child will be attending and ask the administrators to tell you what's required, then submit the form or letter with a letter from your child's endocrinologist (most will have a form letter intended for just this purpose). When you submit the request, be sure to specify that you want a meeting with the administrator(s) and staff in charge of creating and implementing the plan.

By law, the school personnel *must* do the following when notified of a need for a 504 Plan:

- Provide written assurance of nondiscrimination
- Provide notice of nondiscrimination in admission or access to its programs or activities. Notice must be included in a student/parent handbook.
- Designate an employee to coordinate compliance
- Cooperate in providing authorized accommodations
- Request a physician's specific recommendations of needed accommodations
- Request a meeting to discuss 504 Plan and IEP
- Provide grievance procedures to resolve complaints

Your school must set up a meeting with you to discuss the 504 Plan. Understand that school officials probably don't know very much about diabetes care and can't be expected to draw up a plan without your input, so this meeting is likely to be the first of several. You will need to ensure that some form of training is designated for specific individuals who will be supervising your child. At the very least, the teachers and staff all need to be taught to recognize the signs of hypoglycemia and how to treat it—and this is a very bare minimum. It is also key that all teachers and staff are aware that your child *does* need to eat at times not in keeping with the standard meal and snack schedule, and that preventing the child from eating when the child needs to have food (even if it's during class) can have serious consequences to the child's health.

The 504 Plan you're given by your school is not written in stone—you do not *have* to sign, and in fact you *shouldn't* sign it if you feel it doesn't go far enough to protect your child's well being. If the school seems reluctant to do what is necessary, and the 504 Plan is inadequate, you are within your rights to contact a lawyer specializing in disability law to help with the negotiations (see Question 82 for more on this subject). But do keep in mind that once the 504 Plan is signed by all parties, it is a *legally binding contract*. That means you have to do your part, and they have to do theirs.

79. What is a Diabetes Medical Management Plan?

A Diabetes Medical Management Plan (DMMP) is a detailed description of how the school or daycare should handle your child's medical needs while your child is in the care of its staff. It supplies all contact information for parents and healthcare providers; summarizes what the target ranges are, when blood glucose checks should be performed, what the usual doses of insulin are, and when insulin should be given; and outlines what tasks the child is capable of doing alone and what tasks require assistance from staff. It also lists when snacks are to be offered and what supplies must be kept at the school. The DMMP is, in short, a checklist for how the school or daycare staff members are to manage your child's diabetes while the child is in their care.

The DMMP is developed by the child's healthcare team in conjunction with parents and presented to the school personnel who have been designated to supervise the child's care during school hours. The presentation of the DMMP ideally should take place **before the child begins (or returns to) classes** during a meeting that includes parents, the child, the school nurse or other designated staff member(s), and ideally at least one member of the child's diabetes team—that way, any questions, concerns, or confusion can be resolved in a timely fashion.

As the parent, it will be your job to make sure that the DMMP is updated, and school staff alerted to the update, any time the child's regimen changes. You will also need to get into a routine of setting up DMMP meetings with school officials before the start of every school year (we recommend that you set up such meetings **at least** 3 weeks before the start of classes, just as with the 504 Plan requests). It's also a good idea to make contact with the school's nurse or other involved staffers from time to time during the school year—perhaps once a month—to make sure they're implementing the plan correctly, especially if your child's A1c rises within the first two or three months after starting school.

As the parent, it will be your job to make sure that the DMMP is updated, and school staff alerted to the update, any time the child's regimen changes.

80. Who will be monitoring my child's blood sugar and giving insulin injections during the school day?

Ideally, the school nurse and your child's teacher(s) will all be trained in how to recognize the signs of hypoglycemia. The school nurse and at least one other individual *who is always present at the school* must learn how to use a blood glucose meter, how and when to use a glucagon shot, and how to administer insulin. Having someone other than the nurse available to give insulin is important, not only in case the nurse herself is absent from the school because of an illness, but also because some school districts share a school nurse, who may need to go to other schools in the district to care for other students. If this is the situation at your school, you must *insist*—preferably as part of your child's 504 Plan—that someone other than the school nurse be trained to give insulin to your child so that your child's insulin dose is never delayed or omitted because the nurse isn't there.

Because your child's situation requires that personnel at the school be trained in handling diabetes and its complications, it's smart to coordinate a meeting between the persons charged with your child's diabetes care and your diabetes team as part of your 504 Plan development. Your diabetes educator is probably the best person to teach your school's staff how to manage diabetes in a school setting, but as a parent you need to be proactive and make sure that the training takes place. That may mean rattling cages with the school administrators—which can be uncomfortable, but if you aren't an advocate for your child's well-being, it's unlikely anyone else will be!

Be prepared to check up on the school from time to time. Children often will not tell parents of the failure by the school to follow a 504 Plan, out of embarrassment or a desire to "not make waves." It may be up to you to be in contact with the child's teachers or school administrators if you see signs that the plan is not being followed. Abrupt changes in your child's performance, unexpected highs or lows, or a lack of blood glucose meter readings may all be signs that the child's 504 Plan isn't being followed correctly—or that it needs an adjustment.

Elizabeth's comment:

Even though Eric isn't yet in school, I've learned from other parents and from one or two children I've spoken with just how crucial it is that you get the word out to the child's teachers and the school staff. One story really sticks with me. My stepdaughter Kayla, a sophomore in high school, has a friend with Type 1 diabetes. She came home from school one day and told me about a substitute teacher who somehow hadn't gotten the message that there was a special needs student in her class. When the girl got up to go to the nurse to have her blood sugar checked, the substitute teacher tried to prevent her from leaving and accused her of "making it up" so she could ditch class. Although the girl explained that she had diabetes, the teacher didn't know what diabetes was (I was horrified to hear that) and still wouldn't allow the student to leave until Kayla, who had just completed her training on how to care for Eric, spoke up on her behalf and explained why the trip to the nurse was necessary.

After I heard about this, I sent an e-mail to the school's administrators and asked them to check out the story, and—if they weren't already doing so—to make sure that any teacher subbing in that child's class was given information about her health circumstances. I was compelled to do this because I felt that it was unlikely the girl would tell her parents—the experience must have been humiliating and a little scary—and I wanted to make sure the school knew about it so they could correct it. They responded by saying they'd check into the incident, but that subs were generally given a packet of information about these sorts of situations, and this one would be asked for an accounting of why she didn't follow the recommendations.

81. How will having diabetes affect my child's education?

Having diabetes has two impacts on the child's education. First, it means that the child must divide his or her attention, focusing not only on the material being taught but also on the status of his or her blood sugar; and second, it means that your child's school day needs to be structured around meeting the need for food and insulin so that the child's academic performance isn't affected by low or high blood sugars. Low blood sugar affects brain function and makes it difficult to learn or retain new concepts; high blood sugar overloads the brain and can make the child restless or uncomfortable, making it difficult to concentrate and potentially causing the child to become disruptive to the class.

There are also emotional considerations around a diabetes diagnosis that can affect the child's ability to learn and interact appropriately with other children. School-age children newly diagnosed with diabetes may be confused, angry, frightened, depressed, or all of the above (sometimes all at once!), and these feelings will likely affect their blood sugar and, most likely, their performance in class.

TESTING, 1-2-3...

Final exams, college entrance exams, or even run-of-the-mill quizzes and tests are stressful, and the hormones that accompany stress (cortisol and adrenaline) can trigger blood sugar fluctuations in a student with diabetes. Moreover, academic testing can last for hours, and students are often forbidden to have food or drinks in the test room. For this reason, prior arrangements must be made to ensure your child has access to food and insulin when taking tests or final exams. This can be especially important in relation to college entrance exams, such as the PSAT, ACT, or SAT, where the rules regarding what students can bring into the test with them may be restrictive — potentially a huge problem, if the exam administrators aren't notified ahead of time that your child has special health concerns requiring frequent snacks during the test.

Although it's beyond the scope of this book to give a detailed answer on how these factors should be addressed, if they're taken into account and dealt with, there's no reason at all that your child shouldn't be able to perform to the best of his or her ability in school. People with Type 1 diabetes learn just as well as people who don't have diabetes — they simply have to be better organized about how they structure their day so that diabetes considerations don't interfere with learning. The emphasis on organization can actually *improve* your child's ability to learn (as it requires the child to be disciplined in a way that many other children never learn to be), so it's not a bad thing overall.

82. What do I do if my school system is unwilling or unable to work with me to care for my child?

If the school is merely *unwilling*, then your first step is to (politely) explain to them that federal law requires them to assist your child, referring to the statutes listed in Question 77. Be calm, don't get angry, but don't back down. You are legally within your rights to insist that they provide a 504 Plan and stick to it.

Public schools are obligated by federal law to provide a 504 Plan and stick to it.

If they should still drag their feet after being told they're obligated by law to assist you, your next step is to contact the American Diabetes Association's legal advocacy office for advice. A call to their toll-free number (1-800-DIABETES — more contact info is in the Appendix) will get you in touch with a local representative and obtain a packet of information on how to address discrimination — because, make no mistake, a public school's refusal to support your child's education is an illegal act of discrimination. The ADA, according to its web site, "[uses] a four-step process to end discrimination: educate, negotiate, litigate, and legislate." They will help you to educate the school as to why the support is necessary, and assist with negotiations if necessary — and if it comes down to it, they'll even give you advice about taking legal action against the school system.

Suing to obtain your child's rights under the various statutes is not for the faint of heart, however — it can be a prolonged fight, and in the meantime your child's safety and educational well-being may be compromised, which may require you to look at alternatives (see Question 83).

Being *unable* to provide appropriate care for a child with diabetes is a different matter, and more complicated; there are times when budget constraints, state laws, or other obstacles interfere with the ability of the school to provide needed services. In California, for example, the California School Nurses Association and other nursing groups challenged in court the legality of a rule by the state Board of Education that allowed school staff other than nurses to give injections. Although the goal of the lawsuit was to make sure the state couldn't cut costs by firing school nurses, the unintended side effect (when the judge ruled in the nurses' favor) was to leave children with diabetes with no one to give them insulin in school districts where multiple schools shared a nurse. The schools were *willing* to provide care to the children, but they couldn't because they lacked the staff (and had no funds to hire a nurse for every school) — so the schools ended up in the unenviable situation of being required by federal law to provide a service that, because of the state court's ruling and the state's budget problems, they couldn't actually offer.

Here again, working with diabetes advocacy organizations such as the ADA is the best solution — but in a case like this, you should ask the school administrators to work *with* you and the ADA's legal advocates to find a solution. It might be something as simple as having the school request additional funds from the state budget to fulfill the obligation to care for your child, or it may be more complicated than that — a class-action lawsuit, for example, with you and your child among the plaintiffs. Either way, the important factor is reaching out to a source of good legal information and support to help pave the way toward a safe, supportive educational environment for your child.

83. Should I put my child in a private school or try to home-school instead of using the public school system?

Ideally, your decision on how and where your child should be educated should be based on where you think your child will get the best education rather than on anything related to the child's diabetes. Because state and federal laws mandate that school systems accommodate children with special health needs—including diabetes—there is no reason, in theory, why your public school system shouldn't be an appropriate place for your child.

That said, you also need to keep your child's best interests in mind. As we noted in Question 82, not all school systems are equal in terms of funding, staffing, and responsiveness to parents and children's needs. If you feel that the public school system is unwilling or unable to properly manage your child's blood sugar, does not accommodate your child's physical needs, or presents obstacles to your child's ability to learn *in a safe environment*, there's good reason to explore other options.

Keep in mind, however, that unless you can convince a court that the school system is negligent in its treatment of your child or deliberately obstructive to your child's ability to learn and be safe, you'll likely have to pay any costs associated with alternative schooling yourself (although this depends on your state's laws). In our opinion, depending on the circumstances, it may be more effective to try to educate the school staff on the nature of diabetes and its treatment than to fight a pitched battle with a public school system—unless the system is so opposed to (or incapable of) supporting your child that your child's physical safety is at risk, which may be the case if the conflict with the school system is prolonged.

If you're in a situation where home schooling or private schools aren't an option, but your child's health is at risk because of the public school's policies or the staff's attitudes, consult with a lawyer familiar with disability laws about how to approach the matter.

84. Does diabetes cause learning disabilities?

According to the Learning Disabilities Association of America, a true learning disability is a *neurologically based processing problem*. That means that the brain is unable to obtain, interpret, store, or retrieve information — the four basic tasks involved in learning.

While diabetes doesn't actually impair the brain's capability of performing any of these functions, fluctuations in blood glucose (particularly hypoglycemia) can prevent the brain from functioning *well*. For example, if your child's blood glucose is low, he or she may have trouble performing any of these learning-related tasks, simply because the brain lacks the energy from glucose. High blood sugar, on the other hand, doesn't directly impair learning, but the symptoms associated with hyperglycemia could distract your child from the subject at hand, making it harder for the child to retain what's being taught.

If your child is having trouble in school, it may be worthwhile to see if there's any connection between blood glucose levels and performance in the classroom. You may want to arrange with the school to permit monitoring of blood sugar more closely in classes or time periods where your child seems to have greater difficulty learning.

PART SIX

Other Things Parents Worry About

Will my health insurance cover
my child's diabetes care?

What do I do if my insurer denies
one of my claims?

Can my child be denied insurance coverage
for having a preexisting condition?

More . . .

FINANCIAL CONCERNS

85. *Will my health insurance cover my child's diabetes care?*

The answer to this question, unfortunately, is "it depends"—on what type of health insurance coverage you have, on the laws of your state, on whether the policy was in effect and paid up at the time of diagnosis, and on what treatment protocol your child is given. Even the frequency of office visits can influence whether your insurance company is willing to pay for certain expenses. Although the recently passed Affordable Health Care bill should spur some changes in the way insurers process claims, past experience dealing with these issues makes us pessimistic that such changes will happen quickly or easily.

As a result, we recommend that parents learn to be vigilant about insurance as soon as possible. As soon as you're able to after your child's diagnosis, it's worth sitting down with your insurance policy and going through the coverage to see what is covered and what isn't. If you have difficulty determining what's covered and what isn't, contact your insurance agent or call the company's help line and ask.

Dealing with insurance and billing issues will, unfortunately, become a fact of life—an obstacle course that you need to be organized and tenacious to navigate successfully. We can't stress too much how important it is to keep good records from the day of diagnosis onward. Keep track of how many times you test, how much insulin you give (and when you give it), the frequency of visits to your endocrinologist, the A1c results, and any instances of illness your child experiences, particularly if they are diabetes-related. Ideally, you can get specific documentation of A1c results and your endocrinologist's notes from each visit to support your claim. These details will be useful in supporting claims offered to your insurance company.

Elizabeth's comment:

Insurance was a nightmare from day one. Eric was insured under his father's policy, a catastrophic policy that covered nothing but emergency care. It paid for the ER visit and about 60% of the hospital bills, but it didn't cover supplies or follow-up visits to the endocrinologist at all—I thought his diabetes would bankrupt us! The only solution was to switch him to my more comprehensive insurance (which I got through my job), and once the exclusion period passed, that's exactly what I did.

But while having Eric on a comprehensive policy helped a lot in terms of how much I had to pay out of pocket, it didn't make everything all better. For one thing, the new insurer demanded evidence that Eric had been insured for 12 months prior to starting on my policy—our state law required that insurers support pre-existing conditions when someone switches policies if the person insured had been covered by insurance at the time of the diagnosis, and if he had at least a year of coverage prior to switching policies. Thankfully, Eric's dad's policy had been in effect for 13 months at the time of his diagnosis, but I had to really dig into my records to prove that—and the only reason I could was that I'm a packrat who doesn't throw anything away.

*The two most important lessons that I've learned in the first year of handling Eric's insurance are: **be organized**, and **review and save everything**! That means keeping a file that contains all of his blood glucose logs, the reports from his endocrinologist, invoices from both his pediatrician and his endocrinologist…everything that shows when and how*

Eric has been treated. Even the notices from the insurer that say what claims they've received and how much they're paying get saved—I've gotten to the point where any piece of paper I get from Eric's endocrinologist OR our insurance company is opened immediately and goes straight into a file so I know I have it if I need it. You have to keep records that describe everything you do in detail, just in case you need it when the time comes to make a claim for a change in treatment—starting pump therapy, or continuous glucose monitoring, or whatever it may be.

I'd like to think that the health insurance reform bill that just passed will help alleviate some of this stuff—insurers will have less incentive to try and deny, deny, deny once it's illegal for them to drop coverage based on prior health considerations. But I'm just not hopeful that the industry as a whole will do anything other than try to find new ways to squeeze profits out of consumers, or get rid of customers who aren't profitable, and people with chronic illnesses are a big, fat target when it comes to that.

86. What do I do if my insurer denies one of my claims?

When it comes to claims, you should expect the payment process to become more complicated than you may be used to. You will likely start seeing denials of coverage where before your insurer simply processed all claims without comment. It's important that you do not become discouraged by this change, and it's equally important that you challenge or appeal the denials—even if you're denied more than once. The reason denials work so splendidly for insurers is that people don't go to the trouble of appealing because they assume it's a lost cause. If you're tenacious, your appeal can (and often will) be accepted.

As we noted in the previous question, the best thing you can do is be forearmed against denials with documentation of your child's treatment regimen, A1c results, and daily blood glucose logs. And *all* communications with your insurance company should be documented, even if it's just by taking notes of a phone call or keeping fax confirmations.

Elizabeth's comment:

*We had a huge hassle with our insurance company when we tried to put Eric on an insulin pump. Though the insurer originally approved it with the pump manufacturer, two months later I got a denial letter in which they claimed they had no evidence we'd tried to maintain good control with syringes for at least a month. Now, this was ten months post diagnosis—I wanted to ask them, "What do you **think** we were using all this time, voodoo?"*

The documentation they requested was the same we'd already sent in, but when I tried to find out where it went, I got a fair bit of runaround. The process appealing the denial of coverage was time-consuming and not at all clearly laid out. There were forms they required that they didn't tell us we needed, a letter from Eric's endocrinologist that was "mis-filed"—you name it, we heard it.

I got great advice from people who'd "been there/done that" on www.tudiabetes.org, and I'm passing it on:

Learn your policy. Keep a log of your communications: names of everyone you talk to and the dates and times of the con-versations. Keep fax confirmations too, if you send anything by fax, and save email correspondence. Everything you mail should go certified or registered mail, and you need to keep the certification numbers and return receipts, and make sure each piece of paper that you enclose in the certified mail has the certified mail number on it—this is an important step.

Don't give up… the more times you appeal, the less daunting it is, and the less they mess with you.

Find out ahead of time how your state insurance commission/ governance works, how to report the insurance companies to them for harassment and non-compliance — and then do it. It might seem like it doesn't help, but the fact is, the more complaints the state receives, the more it hurts the insurance companies' bond ratings … and some states even fine insurance companies for doing wrong and give the money (minus the administrative fee) to the insured person who filed the complaint. Most people never bother to learn about this because filing a complaint is a pain, but if more people did it, the "deny everything first" policy of most insurance companies might change.

87. What do I do if insurance doesn't cover the cost of supplies and doctor visits?

Diabetes is a very expensive disease. If you don't have insurance, or if your coverage doesn't pay for supplies and regular visits to the endocrinologist, you need to look for assistance as soon as possible.

Diabetes is a very expensive disease. If you don't have insurance, or if your coverage doesn't pay for supplies and regular visits to the endocrinologist, you need to look for assistance as soon as possible — *before* the drain on your finances starts to put you into serious debt. Your first stop should be to contact your state's Health and Human Services Department to see whether a state social worker can advise you on programs offered by the state that will support your child's healthcare needs.

Second, look into the possibility of obtaining insurance for your child as part of a high-risk pool, as outlined in the 2010 Affordable Care Act. An important provision of the Act was to establish a temporary, subsidized high-risk pool to help protect individuals with disabilities from medical bankruptcy. Although this high-risk pool is intended as "a stop-gap measure that will serve as a bridge to a reformed health insurance marketplace," and it's therefore only in place until 2014, its availability is something that families without insurance should take advantage of while they can.

If the services offered by the state aren't enough to help you afford to buy insulin and you don't have insurance coverage, you may be able to get it free or discounted. Prescription assistance programs run by pharmaceutical companies, and nonprofit organizations that focus on helping chronically ill children, can also help you obtain testing and treatment supplies. There are even organizations that help support the cost of obtaining a refurbished insulin pump and related supplies.

It's also important that you be up front with your child's endocrinologist, diabetes educator, and other specialists on his or her team. It may be embarrassing to say, "I can't afford to take care of my child's bills," but it's better to let the healthcare team know where you stand up front, because they cannot help you if they don't know you need help! Most practitioners understand how parents struggle with the costs if they're not insured, and they will likely be willing to help you find resources to support your child's medical needs.

Many pediatric endocrinologists or hospitals either have someone on staff who can assist you with applying for state and federal aid programs, or they can refer you to a specialist who can assist you. So if you're having trouble affording supplies or care, let your diabetes team know immediately. Remember also that it's to your advantage to ask them to help you, because it means that your child will stay healthier and need fewer visits to the doctor or hospital if you get these resources.

At the same time, though, you will need to keep a very close eye on the invoices you get from your provider(s). Medical billing errors do happen (charging for services you didn't receive, for instance, or charging you twice for the same visit), so reviewing the bills is an essential part of keeping your costs down. This can be confusing, especially if the billing department sends the invoice weeks or months after the visit, but don't be afraid to call the billing office and question an item if you don't recognize it or think it might be an error. It also helps to keep records of when your child has doctor's visits so you can double check that the visit you're charged for actually took place. If your child is given blood tests or other lab work, make sure you know what tests were requested so you can verify that the requested tests are the only ones you're charged for.

The National Diabetes Information Clearinghouse has a thorough listing of sources of financial support for people with diabetes, and it's worth a visit. It's aimed at adults, but some of the resources can be used to find support for your child as well. We list this and other resources in the Appendix.

88. Can my child be denied insurance coverage for having a preexisting condition?

At the time of this writing, the Affordable Care Act of 2010 had just passed. The intent of the bill was to eliminate some of the insurance obstacles faced by people with chronic conditions, including the excessive cost of coverage for people with health issues, limitations on how much lifetime coverage is available, and restrictions on what can be covered based on the presence of a pre-existing health condition.

The immediate result of this legislation has been that insurers can no longer exclude uninsured children from obtaining a policy after a diabetes diagnosis—so if your child didn't have insurance prior to the diabetes diagnosis, you can still get health insurance for him or her. If you currently have insurance, your insurer is forbidden to cut your coverage or drop you or your child from the plan because of the change in your child's health status. Also, if your child is on your insurance but is about to graduate college or turn 23, the new law allows parents to maintain coverage on the child until age 27.

However, it remains to be seen how insurers will respond to the new law—whether they'll obey the spirit of the law, which attempts to make health insurance available (and affordable) to all people regardless of their current health status, or whether they'll find loopholes that allow them to avoid extending coverage to the chronically ill.

If you lose insurance coverage for other reasons (such as job loss), look into Medicaid or S-CHIP programs run by individual states that cover children whose parents can't afford or are unable to insure them. The American Diabetes Association website offers a number of options for children with diabetes (see the Appendix).

89. Can I deduct the costs associated with my child's diabetes care on my taxes?

If you can declare your child as your dependent, you can deduct costs related to your child's diabetes care on your taxes—whatever you pay for out of your own pocket (that is, what's not covered by insurance) is considered a legitimate medical expense that you can write off. Considering that, on average, diabetes costs $12,000 or more *per year* over and above the standard healthcare costs that individuals without diabetes normally pay, it is worthwhile to start submitting itemized deductions even if you currently do not do so. If itemized deductions are something you've never done before, it's worth consulting with a tax professional about it, because this is one way to recoup some of the financial burden the child's illness places on your family.

To submit itemized deductions for your child's care, however, you need to document the expenses. This is another reason why it's important to keep good records—*especially* receipts. Whether it's a co-pay for a regular doctor's visit or a bill from an emergency room visit, you should keep *all* receipts and documentation related to your child's diabetes care. Make a habit of putting all receipts, invoices, and insurance payments into a file—it should contain only the current year's receipts, and it should be separate from the file that documents your child's treatment regimen.

EMOTIONAL AND HEALTH CONCERNS

90. What emotional impact will the diagnosis of diabetes have on my child?

To a certain extent, the emotional impact of a diabetes diagnosis depends on two factors: the child's age at diagnosis and the responses of the people the child is closest to (family and friends).

First, the age factor. In general, older children have a tougher time adjusting than younger children. School-age children and teens may be angry at the abrupt, unwelcome change in their lives because it reduces and constrains their autonomy at a time when they're attempting to expand their independence. Depression is also not uncommon, simply because diabetes can be so overwhelming, day after day. Children diagnosed at a very young age (toddlers/preschoolers) tend to adapt better in the short run, because they have a great deal less sensitivity about being "different" from their peers—and their peers also tend to be much more accepting of the differences that accompany life with diabetes. The novelty of the diagnosis and the new experiences (even the unpleasant ones) can be interesting, even intriguing, to a child as he or she tries to make sense of the changes that have come about. But over time, even children diagnosed as infants become conscious that they are unlike their peers in certain respects, and they may become impatient with, or embarrassed by, the limitations and routines imposed by their condition. At some point, the novelty of diabetes gives way to a realization that the diabetes routine is never-ending—there's no getting away from it, ever. The need to always check blood glucose and count carbs becomes tedious, annoying, and a hassle. And, particularly if there's no one else in the family or the local community with diabetes, the child may feel isolated and lonely, because there's no one who truly understands.

How these feelings manifest depend in part on your child's personality. Some children cover embarrassment with outgoing or even aggressive behavior, while others do as much as possible to downplay or hide their "difference"—but however your child copes, the feelings are there, *especially* among pre-teens and teens.

The responses of family and friends can be more problematic because they can be varied and unpredictable. When it comes to the child's friends, the best suggestion we have is that you gather the five or six children your son or daughter is closest to as soon as possible after the diagnosis and explain very clearly to these children exactly what the problem is and how it's going to affect your child's day-to-day life. Most of the time, children's friends are surprisingly sympathetic and understanding—and if given a simple, clear breakdown about the disease, its consequences, and the symptoms of "trouble" (lows, generally speaking), friends frequently will be not only supportive, but often will intercede to summon help for or even treat a child who is experiencing low blood sugar. Another suggestion is to give a presentation to your child's class regarding diabetes so that children better understand—and accept—your child's situation. There are several books written for elementary school children that are intended to be used in this fashion, and we list them in the Appendix.

Other family members' responses to the diagnosis (and, eventually, the way they handle the day-to-day routine that emerges) will also affect the child's emotional response. Many children, even those very young at diagnosis, will likely recall certain aspects about the day of diagnosis—and their parents' emotional responses (tears, expressions of fear or panic) are among the factors that tend to stick with the child most. Such memories aren't necessarily the most significant factor affecting children's responses, however—what's more important is how family members adjust to the undeniably traumatic and stressful transition from diabetes crisis to diabetes routine. Parents who adjust well, who learn to accept the changes, and who manage the disease as just another part of the family routine make it easy for children to do the same. Parents who fuss, nag, and show non-stop anxiety over diabetes care increase the child's stress and make it more likely that the child will rebel or become depressed. This is especially true if fussing and nagging become a substitute for warmth and affection.

If you recognize yourself as a "nagger" with anxiety as your primary emotion regarding your child's condition, please understand that you're hardly alone—and that our description is not intended as a criticism. Parents who love their child and care about the child's health naturally are inclined to fuss and worry, and it's *very* hard to stifle the impulse! Our intention here is not to point fingers, but to make parents aware how important it is to be conscious of their behavior. There will be times when nagging is necessary to make sure your child stays healthy and safe, but there will be other times when you'll need to learn to bite your tongue and back off. This is especially important (and difficult) when the time comes to let your child take the lead in his or her own care. If you find yourself spending more time feeling and acting anxious or controlling, or if you're continually fighting with your child about his or her diabetes care, it's time to call for help from your diabetes team or a counselor who understands the issues involved with diabetes.

Of course, parents aren't the only family members involved. Siblings, grandparents, and other extended family who interact with the child can affect the child's emotional welfare significantly. Siblings may be jealous of the attention given the child with diabetes, or of the fact that their brother or sister can eat "anything they want, any time they want, even in school"—generally not realizing that it's not a matter of choice or preference. Alternatively, siblings might mimic their parents' expressions of worry and anxiety, inadvertently becoming a source of irritation when they follow the parents' lead and nag, hover, or try to control their brother or sister. Grandparents, likewise, can add to the child's stress if their anxiety about the child's health leads them to either fuss over the child or distance themselves from the child. Even expressions of sympathy, if repeated each time the child sees a grandparent or an aunt, can become grating, prompting resentment rather than affection — after all, who wants to constantly be an object of pity?

In most cases, the solution for familial factors is education, both informal and formal. Informally, relatives who are prone to expressing anxiety or pity, or who avoid the child with diabetes during family get-togethers, should be taken aside and gently corrected so their response doesn't become another burden for an already overburdened child to carry. From a more formal standpoint, siblings and grandparents should be made more comfortable about the child's condition by learning about it — whether through books, classes, or videos — so they can understand that, while diabetes is a reality that all family members need to be aware of, it is not a rationale for treating the child differently than they otherwise would. The more other family members understand about your child's diabetes, the easier it will be for your child to adjust emotionally to the reality of living with diabetes.

91. How do I cope with the stress this diagnosis has put on my family?

Although individuals and families cope with stress in their own unique ways, there are certain things you can do (and other things you should avoid doing) to help reduce the stress of managing your child's diabetes.

First, keep in mind that your family has experienced a traumatic loss. Your child's health status is unalterably changed, and that fact will be *the* dominant factor in your daily life for the first few weeks or months until you develop a stable routine for managing the child's diabetes. Even after diabetes is no longer new and frightening, it will be a constant in your life—sometimes an unwelcome constant. It is normal and acceptable to feel grief, anger, or sadness over your child's condition, and you should allow yourself to acknowledge these feelings once the initial emergency of the diagnosis has passed. We strongly suggest that parents and other family members, including older siblings, grandparents, and extended family take the time to talk about what the diagnosis means for your child, for you, and for the rest of the immediate family.

It is normal and acceptable to feel grief, anger, or sadness over your child's condition.

Second, recognize that the diagnosis of diabetes in your child probably brings with it a very high dose of fear for everyone involved—you, your child, your child's siblings and friends, and other family members outside of the immediate household. The best antidote to fear is knowledge. We are far less frightened by what we know than by something unfamiliar. Learn everything you can about your child's health circumstances and be ready, willing, and able to teach your child(ren), your relatives, other caregivers, and even your child's friends what the diagnosis really means in a matter-of-fact and reassuring way. And understand that this is not going to be something you can do in a week, or even a month!

Third, make connections with other families who have children with diabetes. Not only will you learn a lot from the more experienced families who've been dealing with the disease for years longer than you have, but you also may take some comfort in knowing that you're not alone in your stress! In urban areas, there may be support groups that meet on a regular basis; in more rural areas, you may need to turn to online organizations. There are a number of sites that offer chat rooms or online support groups for children as well as parents. We list some of these in the Appendix, but you can also find them by searching the internet using "children with diabetes support groups" or similar search terms.

At the risk of sounding like we're contradicting ourselves, however, it helps no one (and may even be damaging to you, your child, or other family members) if you spend too much time focusing on your trauma. Yes, diabetes has changed your life, your child's life, and the lives of other family members forever, but sooner or later you need to allow your lives to fall back into a normal rhythm. It might be a different rhythm than the one your family had prior to the diagnosis, but it's still a normal rhythm (even if it doesn't feel that way at first). And one of the best ways to get that sense of normality back is to consciously address your emotions. If you find yourself feeling depressed, angry, or just "stuck" in negative feelings, individual or family grief counseling may be appropriate. Talk to your diabetes team, as they may be able to refer you to a counselor who is accustomed to helping families adjust to life's changes after a child is diagnosed with diabetes.

Elizabeth's comment:

In the immediate aftermath of Eric's diagnosis, my husband and I both had to take time to have "mini-meltdowns" over it. My husband went first. About 2 weeks after we left the hospital, he was so grouchy and scatterbrained that I finally e-mailed one of his good friends, a man who'd lived all his life with a chronic disease himself, and said, "Get him out of here!" The friend went straight to our house and asked my husband to join him for the weekend up at his cabin in the woods, ostensibly to help "fix the place up" for hunting season. My husband initially didn't want to go—he felt like he'd be abandoning me to leave me to take care of all three kids alone—but I told him we'd be fine and he went. I don't know what they talked about but he was in a much better frame of mind when he returned.

A month later it was my turn. I had thought I was doing fine, but it just hit me all of a sudden—I started snapping at people and being impatient with the kids, and I wasn't sleeping well, so finally one day my husband simply told me to go spend the night at my mother's and take a mini-vacation. I needed the break, that much was clear, and while I was away I decided I needed to connect with other parents somehow. We live in a small town in Maine, so the internet seemed the obvious solution. I found a couple of diabetes-oriented social networking sites and started blogging about my experience and troubles, and the interaction with other parents and people with diabetes has been very, very helpful to me. I honestly don't know how I'd have managed this past year without this community.

92. How can I be sure I won't harm my child by mistake?

Elizabeth's comment:

The best advice Eric's endocrinologist ever gave us was something he said as we were leaving the hospital. He said, "Don't try to be his pancreas. You're not his pancreas. You're his parents." What he meant was (and I didn't figure this out until several months later) that we weren't going to be able to keep Eric in perfect control all the time, and there would be times we'd screw up royally. As parents, we want to do the best we can for our children, but we're human beings — we're going to make mistakes. This was brought home to me force- fully one night when I inadvertently gave Eric more than twice the amount of Lantus [long-acting insulin] he needed. Fortunately, I realized my mistake and called the diabetes clinic immediately. Then I had a complete emotional melt- down. I had visions of having to go to the emergency room and potentially having Eric in the ICU again — even imag- ined a horrible scenario where the Department of Human Services weighed in on whether I was fit to raise a child with diabetes! — but it turned out that all I needed to do was make sure he got 20 carbs an hour for the next 24 hours. And though that was certainly no fun, it wasn't nearly as bad as had I feared. I felt pretty foolish afterward that I'd gotten so distraught, but the first time you make a mistake, it's easy to blow it out of proportion.

That experience taught me two things: first, when dealing with Eric's insulin, I needed to deal ONLY with Eric's insu- lin and put all other considerations aside. The mistake had happened because I was tired from a long day at work, fight- ing with my teenage stepdaughter, and trying to make dinner for myself at the same time I was drawing up the insulin. That's too many tasks for a stressed-out parent's brain! And second, I learned not to panic when I make a mistake — had I stopped to think about it, I'd have realized that even so- called rapid-acting insulin doesn't take effect right away, so an overdose (even a massive one) is not going to immedi- ately shoot the child into a life-threatening low, and chances are good that it can be corrected within the time frame of the insulin's action — especially if you've got juice, chocolate syrup, or a glucagon shot readily available, all of which we had. So my advice to parents is, allow yourself to be human, and accept that you're going to make a mistake sooner or later. You and your child will be better off for it.

Ultimately, it's not very likely that you'll harm your child in the course of treating his or her diabetes. Accidents happen, people make mistakes, but if you are conscientious, focused, and keep in close contact with your diabetes educator and clinic staff, none of these are likely to be very serious problems. Moreover, as Elizabeth notes, even an insulin overdose isn't likely to have an immediate impact on your child's blood sugar—and if you do accidentally give your child too much insulin, the glucagon kit can be used to counteract the insulin (and glucagon *does* have an immediate effect!)

Accidentally harming your child while treating him or her isn't the greatest danger in diabetes. The greater danger is what happens if you DON'T treat it, or if you're reluctant or fearful about managing it. Untreated or poorly treated diabetes is *guaranteed* to harm your child—maybe not immediately, but certainly over the long run. The most damage you could do as a parent would be imparting to your son or daughter the feeling that diabetes is something to be ignored, or feared, or set aside because you just don't feel like dealing with it. Your child will follow your lead when it comes to handling his or her diabetes, so if you're fearful or ambivalent about it, your child will be too—and over the years, that is what's going to prevent him or her from maintaining good blood glucose control, which is where those dreaded complications come in (which we'll describe in detail in Question 93).

It can be difficult to set aside your emotions about the diabetes diagnosis and treatment. If you find yourself having such difficulties, we encourage you to talk with your diabetes educator or a social worker familiar with the issues of raising a child with diabetes. Suppressing your fears (or denying you have them) is the worst thing a parent can do, because your child will inevitably pick up on your feelings and will probably imitate them.

93. What are the long-term complications of diabetes, and can I prevent them?

ALL of the complications associated with diabetes ARE PREVENT-ABLE.

We'll give you the good news first: ***ALL of the complications associated with diabetes ARE PREVENT-ABLE.*** We intentionally put that message in boldface, capital letters, and italics because it's crucial that you, as a parent, understand that none of this is inevitable. The complications of diabetes are enough to scare the willies out of any parent, but you shouldn't let them—instead, use them as motivation to do the best job you can (and teach your child likewise) in maintaining good control.

So, on to the bad news. You've undoubtedly already heard frightening stories about some of the complications related to diabetes: blindness, kidney failure, heart disease, nerve damage, and limb amputation. What these boil down to, in essence, is damage done to blood vessels by the excess sugar in the blood. When blood sugar is consistently high over long periods of time, the sugar molecules attach to proteins in the blood and alter them so that they don't function properly. Blood vessels become thicker and less elastic, which makes the pressure of the blood in the vessel higher. The blood vessels may become scarred and blocked (**atherosclerosis**), or may develop leaks, particularly within the kidneys. Tiny capillaries that feed the skin, nerves, and eyes are among the first to suffer damage, but over the course of years, even larger blood vessels feeding the major organs, particularly the heart, can become injured too.

Atherosclerosis

Hardening and blockage of arteries.

Atherosclerosis is the culprit in the heart disease and strokes that are a concern in adults with diabetes; kidney failure results from the damage done to renal blood vessels over time. In the eyes, blood vessel changes can lead to a condition called **retinopathy** that, if not addressed, eventually leads to distortion of the retina and loss of sight. Nerve damage, skin infections, and worst of all limb amputations are all related to impaired blood flow as well.

Retinopathy
Damage to the eye that distorts the retina and leads to vision loss in people with diabetes.

All of this sounds rather grim, but you need to keep perspective about it. It takes years, even decades, of very poor control for diabetes complications to develop. That means that your child has a fair amount of time to work on gaining control over his or her blood sugar to avoid these problems, and it can be done. A study in 1993 called the Diabetes Control and Complications Trial (DCCT) showed that when people with Type 1 diabetes tested more frequently and worked to maintain a near-normal blood glucose level ("tight control," as described in Question 27), they had far fewer complications than those who didn't.

It's very clear from this study and others that preventing complications really depends on keeping overall blood glucose stable. The equation is pretty simple. The less excess glucose floating around in the blood stream, the less opportunity there is for glucose to fuse to blood proteins and cause damage to the blood vessels. At the same time, though, you don't want to overdo it and keep blood glucose *too* low, since that's what leads to hypoglycemia and all the problems related to that condition. So it's a balancing act. Keep blood glucose low enough to avoid blood vessel damage, while maintaining it high enough to prevent hypoglycemia.

This is where the hemoglobin A1c test we talked about in Question 22 comes in. Over time, researchers looking at diabetes complications have found that the A1c is a pretty good indicator of the likelihood of long-term health problems. A1c, as you may recall from the earlier discussion, measures the average blood glucose level over a period of about three months. Keeping tabs on your child's A1c is, therefore, a great way to monitor the stability of the child's overall blood glucose.

Ideally, an A1c below 7% is what you're looking for — although remember that lower isn't necessarily better if it comes at the cost of regular episodes of hypoglycemia! And keep in mind that an A1c of 7% or lower isn't always easy (or possible) to achieve in children; as we mentioned earlier, with very young children who get insulin injections after they eat, it's very difficult to obtain an A1c below 8%, and in teens, we usually see higher A1c values for a variety of reasons. However, even slight reductions in A1c values can mean significant reductions in risk of complications, so any decrease in the A1c, no matter how small, is something to cheer.

There are other factors that can help reduce the risk of individual complications as well. For example, studies in African Americans with Type 1 diabetes showed that a low calorie, low sodium diet substantially reduced progression of retinopathy. Regular visits to an eye specialist familiar with diabetes are also an important step in preventing eye damage. Likewise, good oral hygiene and regular dental care can prevent not only the complications of tooth loss, but also certain oral infections that can lead to higher blood sugars, such as candidiasis (yeast infection of the mouth). And another important area for prevention is the skin, which is prone to infections and sores in people with diabetes. Keeping skin clean and moisturized, and quickly treating dry skin, rashes, or inflamed areas to prevent them from developing into infections, can help your child avoid complications.

It probably goes without saying that avoiding tobacco and alcohol are of critical importance to limiting complications as your child grows into adulthood. We're all aware that both of these substances have profound health effects on people even without diabetes, and naturally the damage they do is only magnified by diabetes. Alcohol, in particular, can be a killer for people with diabetes because alcohol can cause low blood sugar, while simultaneously making the person drinking it unaware that he or she is experiencing a low—particularly if he or she drinks to excess and becomes unconscious. Making it plain that smoking and drinking are off limits because of diabetes may be something that won't sit well with teens, but it's a subject that parents should address head on (and it may mean reducing or eliminating your own use of tobacco or alcohol so as not to seem like a hypocrite—and more practically, to make it more difficult for your teens to get their hands on either one!)

> *It probably goes without saying that avoiding tobacco and alcohol are of critical importance to limiting complications as your child grows into adulthood.*

94. At what age is it okay to start talking to my child about diabetes complications?

One question that often comes up with parents is how and when to tell the child about these complications. That's one of those classic unanswerable questions; it really depends on your child's personality and how fast he or she matures.

What you *don't* want to do is overload the child with frightening information before he or she is ready—it will only make the child feel hopeless, depressed, or anxious, and none of these emotions help with good diabetes control. But at the same time, it's also not a good idea to try to hide the truth about complications from your child. In the internet era, all the child needs to do is search on "diabetes complications" to learn all the gory details, but there's a pretty good chance that the information that pops up on the screen may be inaccurate, out of date, or not applicable to your child at all (and most children don't know how to distinguish good information from bad). Without parental guidance, learning about all the horrible things that *could* happen might be pretty traumatic — so it's best if you make sure that you're available to act as both teacher and comforter when the time comes for your child to come face to face with the full picture of what diabetes can mean.

In general, the best strategy we've found is to educate your child on what diabetes means for day-to-day life in a matter-of-fact way, let the child know in general terms that good diabetes control will prevent certain health problems later in life, and leave it to your child's discretion to ask about those health problems when he or she is ready to learn more.

When you do discuss the matter, remember to stress the message we talked about in Question 93. None of the complications or health problems you're talking about is inevitable, and with good self-care and tight control of blood glucose over the long term, your child can expect to live a long, healthy life.

95. Are there any other diseases that a child with diabetes might be prone to?

Yes. In essence, the Type 1 diabetes diagnosis is a sign that your child's immune system is prone to overreact against the body's own cells, and as a result, your child may be at higher risk of developing certain other auto-immune disorders somewhere down the line. The two most common are celiac disease, which we mentioned briefly in Question 55, and autoimmune thyroid disorders. Other, less common autoimmune diseases include Addison's disease (autoimmune dysfunction of the adrenal glands), a skin disorder called vitiligo, and a neurological disorder called myasthenia gravis.

Pediatric endocrinologists commonly recommend that children be screened periodically for celiac and thyroid disease.

Celiac Disease

Celiac disease is an autoimmune disorder that stems from exposure to gluten in certain foods (we describe these foods in Question 55). In the general population, roughly 1 person in 100 develops celiac, but among people with Type 1 diabetes, that number is closer to 1 in 8 or 1 in 10 — different studies offer slightly different estimations, but the point is, celiac is almost 10 times more common in people with autoimmune diabetes. Your child may not have it at the time the diabetes is diagnosed, but it may develop later, so it's something to watch for.

Although the "classic" symptoms of celiac disease include chronic bowel problems (diarrhea or constipation), abdominal pain, gas, and bloating, your child may not have these symptoms yet still have celiac. As odd as it may seem when we're talking about an autoimmune reaction in the intestines, children with celiac sometimes have symptoms that are completely unrelated to digestion—or no symptoms at all!

Even without symptoms, celiac is a serious problem that can greatly affect your child's overall well-being and prevent you from obtaining good control of the child's diabetes. If you're told your child has celiac, it is important that your child starts to avoid gluten entirely, because even with no symptoms, celiac disease is very damaging to your child's digestive system. The intestinal damage done by celiac in turn affects the child's ability to digest and absorb food—resulting in unstable blood sugar levels and even malnutrition! In children with diabetes, a pattern of unexplained lows is often the very first sign of the development of celiac disease.

Your child should be periodically tested for celiac even if there are no symptoms, but it's especially important to ask your pediatrician or endocrinologist to order a test if your child has headaches, generalized joint or bone aches, fatigue, skin rashes, or other seemingly disconnected complaints. It may also be worthwhile taking your child off gluten for a couple of weeks (that is, having him or her completely avoid anything made with wheat, rye, or barley flour—what's called an "elimination diet" in allergy circles) to see if any such symptoms go away. If they do, your child may have celiac, or may simply have a milder sensitivity to gluten—try reintroducing gluten-containing foods a little at a time to see if symptoms come back. If they do, discuss this problem with your physician.

Autoimmune Thyroid Disease

The thyroid is a gland in your neck that produces hormones that regulate metabolism. Many people with Type 1 diabetes also develop an autoimmune disorder of the thyroid, but it is a frustrating subject for doctors to talk about with parents and patients because there is no data showing the prevalence of thyroid problems in Type 1 diabetes (current estimates in the medical literature puts it at 15%–20%).

Because of this, most children with Type 1 diabetes are screened yearly for thyroid function. There are two types of thyroid problems that can develop: low thyroid function (autoimmune hypothyroidism, also known as Hashimoto's thyroiditis), and hyperthyroidism (Graves' disease), in which the thyroid over-produces its hormones. Hashimoto's is far more common than Graves' in children with diabetes.

There are certain symptoms parents can watch for that can alert them to have their child screened for thyroid function, including:

- unusual fatigue that is not related to out-of-range blood sugars
- constipation
- dry skin, dull or brittle hair, or thinning eyebrows
- sensitivity to cold, including feeling cold in a room at normal room temperature (68° F), or feeling numbness or a painful prickling in fingers or toes on a cold day, or a cold-related rash or hives that disappears when warmth is applied
- menstrual irregularities
- muscle weakness
- hoarse voice

Fortunately, treating hypothyroidism is pretty simple. There are several forms of synthetic thyroid hormones on the market, including Synthroid and Levoxyl. The main difficulty is keeping the dose adjusted to your child's needs as the child grows, which is why regular thyroid checks will be necessary if your child is diagnosed with hypothyroidism.

96. How do I teach my child to take diabetes seriously and do what's necessary to stay healthy?

Teaching your child about diabetes is a tight-rope walk. On the one hand, you want them to understand that it's serious, it's important, and it's something they need to pay close attention to if they're to stay healthy. On the other hand, you don't want them to be afraid or anxious, or to feel that diabetes limits their ability to enjoy life, learn new things, or have fun. How do parents find the happy medium between impressing the sometimes grim and frightening facts upon their child without scaring the heck out of them?

If you want your child to grow up being aware, but not anxious, about diabetes, then you need to train yourself to have this attitude first.

To a certain extent, this is accomplished by first training yourself. If you want your child to be consistent and responsible in managing diabetes care, then you first must make sure that *you* are consistent and responsible. If you want your child to thoroughly understand how to take care of his or her diabetes, you have to do your homework first so that you can teach these essentials. And if you want your child to grow up being aware, but not anxious, about diabetes, then you need to train yourself to have this attitude first. This may seem unimaginable to a parent of a newly diagnosed child, but remember—*you're not alone in this.* Thousands of other parents have been where you stand now; thousands more will follow. You can learn a lot by talking to adults with Type 1 diabetes as well as parents of children with Type 1 diabetes—and a lot of what they have to tell you will help you to teach your child, in turn.

Children will follow their parents' lead, and they're quick to note contradictions. If you tell your child "there's nothing to be afraid of," but are constantly betraying your own anxieties by hovering, your child is going to understand that there *is* something to fear, and that you're simply not being honest. On the other hand, you also don't want to hold the threat of complications over your child's head to make him or her more compliant with the diabetes regimen. In practical terms, "You'd better do X or not do Y, or you could go blind" is completely useless as a threat once the child tests it and finds that, in fact, his or her eyesight is perfectly fine after doing (or not doing) X or Y—unlike parents, children tend to see things in terms of immediate, rather than long-term, results. And from the standpoint of your relationship with the child, what the child perceives is that you are willing to exaggerate the truth or even lie outright in order to get obedience—because, even though the possibility of blindness is a real one, children don't think in terms of what's going to happen in 30 or 40 years, so if blindness doesn't strike immediately, they again conclude you're being dishonest. Where diabetes is concerned, as with anything, it's best that you maintain open and honest dialogue with your child.

At the same time, you also need to realize that sooner or later, your child is going to need to learn to deal with diabetes personally. You, as a parent, can offer guidance, but you can't dictate how your child will come to terms with what is, at least at present, a life-long circumstance.

Nagging, harassing, and hassling come all too easily to parents, but they aren't helpful; talk, support, and making sure your child feels secure, loved, and able to trust you are of key importance.

Here again, both you and your child can learn from others' experiences. Meeting other children of the same age through support groups, online or otherwise, or at diabetes camps can make a world of difference to how well children learn to manage their diabetes. And talking with other parents can help *you* to learn better parenting skills, both around diabetes and overall. We can't stress too strongly how important it can be for both you *and* your child that you reach out to others who know what you're going through.

It probably wouldn't hurt your child to interact with some adults with Type 1 diabetes through online communities, either. Diabetes care has changed substantially over the decades, and the stories told by men and women diagnosed 20, 30, even 40 years ago can be amazing and instructive ... as well as encouraging. Many of these individuals have survived against much more difficult obstacles and much greater odds than your child will face—with a great deal less support and reason to hope for an eventual cure than your child now has. Learning from those who've gone before may help your child to realize just how fortunate he or she really is—and how manageable diabetes can be with comparatively little effort (once you all know the ropes!).

Elizabeth's comment:

I owe a lot of what I've learned in the past year to online communities and books written by other parents, and sometimes by talking to people who've lived with Type 1 diabetes for

30 years or more. Since Eric is only 3, I don't have any experience with older children who have diabetes—but I have raised my two teenage stepchildren, so I'm pretty familiar with how the school-age and adolescent mind works. It's a roller-coaster ride even without diabetes in the mix! A book that I think is particularly useful is Getting a Grip on Diabetes: Quick Tips and Techniques for Kids and Teens, *written by Spike and Bo Loy. These two young men—brothers who were diagnosed when they were in elementary school—have put together a fairly comprehensive guide addressing issues that teens explore while making the transition from child to adult. It talks about athletics, school, college, even alcohol and drug use . . . everything except sex, which I guess they didn't get into because it wouldn't be gentlemanly. It's advanced enough that parents should probably screen it before giving it to the teenager—the sort of thing you should read and discuss with your child instead of just handing it off—but it's very, very useful and probably will mean more because it comes from two young men who have "been there, done that." It's unbelievably pragmatic and practical, and it seems like that's really what children need to learn in order to navigate diabetes well.*

97. Will my child resent me for having to constantly prick him with needles? Will my child blame me for all the difficulties and restrictions that go with diabetes?

No child wants to be given injections, but many parents are even more opposed to the idea of giving them than the child is. This is, of course, only natural, as parents understand that their role in life is to protect, rather than hurt, their children. It runs counter to every instinct we have as parents to stick needles in our kids' skin!

In many respects, your child's attitude toward your giving injections will reflect two factors: first, the child's age and ability to comprehend what having diabetes really means, and second, what he or she sees in your own attitude.

Young children (0 to 7 years old)

For very young children, meaning infants and toddlers through, roughly, first graders, injections may mean confusion at first—the child simply doesn't understand why Mommy or Daddy keeps "hurting" them all the time. At the same time, though, your child isn't likely to blame you for it. With young children, it's actually more the opposite—they see that their parent is upset, unhappy, or frustrated by their condition, and think *they* have done something wrong. You may feel anger, hostility, guilt, or fear about the fact that your child needs the injection, and it's likely that your child can read these emotions in your body language, or in the things you say out loud (perhaps without even realizing it), while preparing an injection. The child might not realize that these feelings are directed at the *disease* and not at the child him- or herself, and so may internalize the idea that you somehow dislike or disapprove of him or her. This mistaken idea may even be heightened by the fact that injections *hurt*—and lead the child to feel that you're giving the injection as punishment, rather than as something intended to make your child healthy.

One way to minimize this issue is to make a point of becoming highly proficient at giving injections without hitting muscle (which is considerably more painful than subcutaneous injections) and choosing sites carefully to maximize the "padding" between the needle and sensitive nerve endings.

It's important in this phase that you talk matter-of-factly and in simple, clear terms to explain to your child that the injections aren't about punishment, and that even if Mom or Dad gets upset, *you're not upset at your child.* The child needs to know more than anything that you are giving injections out of love, so that you can keep them healthy and feeling well. If the child is old enough to recognize symptoms of highs and lows, those sensations can be used to clarify the purpose of the injections. "Remember when you had that terrible headache and felt really nauseous, and I found out your blood sugar was high? I gave you the insulin injection and you felt better—that's what insulin is for."

School-age children

With older kids, you need to watch out for misinformation, which is one of the prime sources of emotional upheaval between you and your child. School children have an amazing wealth of myths, fallacies, errors, and down-right lies that they pass on to one another—these days, at the speed of a text message—and your child will unques-tionably be fed some of these at some point. For example, your child might "learn" from another kid at school that the diabetes diagnosis came from eating too many sweets, because "only fat kids who eat a lot of junk food get diabe-tes!" (or words to that effect). The (erroneous) notion that diabetes is caused by too much sugar and too little exer-cise is pervasive in the public mindset, and it's very likely that your child will confront this myth before very long. Exposure to this kind of garbage information can breed feelings of resentment and anger, so it's important to keep the information flow positive, not only so that your child can understand that such accusations aren't true, but also so that your child has the ability to correct the perpetra-tor's ignorance—which can be very empowering.

But the older a child is, the more he or she might be prone to having difficult emotions about the diagnosis. *Why me?* is a question most people, whether adults or children, ask themselves when struck with a condition as difficult and frightening as diabetes, and *why me?* is frequently followed by an attempt to pin the blame on someone. If it's clear to the child that he or she didn't do anything to "deserve" diabetes (and for the sake of full disclosure, we should note that it often *isn't* clear to the child that diabetes isn't punishment for some imagined or hidden mistake), then the next person likely to be singled out for blame is (you guessed it) Mom or Dad, or maybe both. Parents are easy targets, after all—they're jointly responsible for the child's genes, they were the source of all food while the child was growing up, they chose the house, daycare, school, neighborhood, city, state, even country where the child was raised—in the mind of a child, parents are in charge of the universe. So how can they not be responsible for the child's diabetes? Reason enough to resent the persons giving the injections (even if your child has already taken over that task, it's generally still the parent who is "making" them inject insulin!).

The solution to these feelings and resentments is to continually maintain a dialogue with your child about diabetes and the feelings he or she has toward the diagnosis. The child needs to truly understand that his or her condition is *nobody's fault*—that it's a complicated intersection of any number of factors that no single person could control. At the same time, though, remember that even with perfect comprehension of this fact, your child may still have feelings of anger, guilt, sadness, and resentment because he or she must live with this disease—especially once your child realizes that diabetes will be in his/her life *forever.* These feelings are a) 100% normal and b) not restricted to children—adults who've lived all their lives with diabetes have them too! The key point is that the child needs to be able to express these feelings to you and know that you're not going to get defensive, angry, or distant in response. It may be tough to keep yourself from reacting in any of those ways when your child is acting hostile, or even openly blaming you for his or her condition—but remind yourself continually that you should not take it personally. Whatever things your child might do or say—and children sometimes say absolutely *awful* things to parents under these circumstances—remember that what they're really mad at isn't you, it's the disease.

Of course, this doesn't mean you have to put up with never-ending abuse, particularly if it devolves into physical abuse. If your child's emotional upset creates such stress and chaos in your life that you find yourself having difficulty with day-to-day functioning, then it's time to call for help—a family counselor familiar with diabetes, or a member of your diabetes team may be an appropriate starting point.

Children sometimes say absolutely awful things to parents under these circumstances—remember that what they're really mad at isn't you, it's the disease.

98. Is there any possibility that my other children will also develop diabetes?

Although it is possible that another of your children will develop Type 1 diabetes, the good news is that it's highly unlikely. Studies of children with diabetes have shown that only about 6% have siblings who are also diagnosed with diabetes. The rate is somewhat higher if one or both parents also has diabetes, particularly if the parent with diabetes is the father.

Clinical trials are currently testing parents and siblings of children with Type 1 diabetes to identify whether other members of the family have autoantibodies or other markers that could show they're at risk for developing the disease themselves. If you're worried about other children in your family, it would probably be a good idea to see if you can join one of these trials. The TrialNet Natural History Study, for example, is a large-scale trial currently underway in a number of countries. In the United States, you can find out more by going to the web site of the National Institute of Diabetes and Digestive and Kidney Diseases (NIDDK). We include information about this trial in the Appendix.

As much as parents find it difficult and stressful to think about their other children developing diabetes, it can actually be beneficial for a child with diabetes to experience a sibling's diagnosis and treatment. When two or more children in a family have diabetes, it puts them all on an equal playing field. The child with diabetes is no longer the "different" one who gets all the special attention (or restrictions) because of his or her illness. Siblings with diabetes have an automatic source of support. Their brother or sister knows *exactly* what they're going through, even when other family members just "don't understand." So while no one would ever wish to have a second child develop diabetes, if yours does, there may be a few silver linings in it for you—not only will you already be experienced in what to do, but also, the first sibling to have diabetes will be able to help the second (and eventually, vice versa).

99. How do I cope with my teenager's rebellion against diabetes?

One endocrinologist sums up the care of teens with diabetes this way: "You just try to get them through it [adolescence] alive." Adolescence is the phase of development when children try to separate themselves from their parents, test their limits, and explore their identity. And it's often the case that diabetes is one of the aspects that the child seeks to set aside, particularly if the bulk of the diabetes management in the child's life has been undertaken by the parent. At the same time, this is a period of physical development marked by hormone-related high blood sugars, particularly first thing in the morning (so-called **dawn phenomenon**), so that even adolescents who are diligent about their diabetes care will have less control than you might like.

Your best strategy at a time like this might be to encourage your child to interact more with other teens who have diabetes, whether that be through an online chat room, in a support group, or at a diabetes camp (see Question 74). Adolescents tend to value the opinions and input of their peers far more than that of their parents. Enlisting the help of other friends, with or without diabetes, in steering your child toward taking more responsibility for his or her health can also be helpful. What comes across as nagging from a mother or father is far more effective when it comes from the mouth of the kid from down the block who's been your child's best friend since grade school.

Parents may be frustrated and confused when children who seemed to understand the importance of checking blood sugar and keeping snacks available appear to "forget" what they've known how to do since third grade. Lecturing them and trying to "re-teach" what they already know will get you a lot of eye-rolling and silent fuming, but it isn't likely to make them more responsible. Bear in mind that this is a stage of growth and that all teens go through this phase in one way or another, and do what you can to set limits without being constrictive. That may mean negotiating diabetes care as a prerequisite for privileges.

Dawn phenomenon

High blood sugars observed early in the morning, most often seen in teenagers because of the pattern of growth hormone release.

Here's an example. Your teenage son asks to borrow the car so he can take his girlfriend out to the movies (she doesn't drive). He hasn't been all that responsible about keeping snacks handy and has recently had some nasty episodes of hypoglycemia because of it, and you don't like the idea of him driving. The easiest way to ensure his safety is to refuse permission, but a couple of alternatives are to a) allow him to drive on the condition that he take his blood glucose and eat a snack in your presence just before he leaves, or b) allow him to go, and give him money to pay for the movie and snacks, but drive them yourself and set a time to pick them up. Or, set a rule that your son's ability to drive himself is dependent upon his A1c value remaining at or below a level specified by the diabetes team, and that his most recent A1c value determines whether you drive or he drives (and if he drives, he still must take his blood sugar and eat in your presence). Either option is going to be difficult for your son to accept, as they both imply that you distrust his judgment—but if he hasn't shown himself to use good judgment, why should you trust it? When it comes to your child's safety, don't feel guilty and don't give in! But try to be matter-of-fact and dispassionate when you explain these realities, because once it turns into a fight, you've lost any leverage you might have had in directing him toward more responsible behavior.

For children diagnosed with diabetes in the teen years, accepting the changes diabetes brings is going to be very hard. Getting the child into counseling and encouraging engagement with other teens who've had diabetes longer are probably the two most valuable steps a parent can take. But even for children who've lived with diabetes for years, adolescence can be rough. Parents should expect that their teen's A1c values and overall diabetes control probably will be worse than when he or she was younger.

Expect, also, that diabetes may become a point of conflict between you and your child during the teen years. Factors such as sexual activity, alcohol use, and drug use are also going to loom large, given that these will have an impact on diabetes control as well (never mind that these factors tend to be sources of parental angst even without adding diabetes into the equation). In girls, the stereotypical obsession with weight and body image is particularly dangerous because girls with Type 1 diabetes are prone to eating disorders, so keep a sharp eye out for signs of ketoacidosis or rapid changes in her weight.

All of this is normal, and it's no fun for parents—but sooner or later your child will realize that there are fewer unpleasant symptoms to contend with and that life, overall, runs more smoothly when he or she maintains good blood glucose control. Until that realization occurs, you're just going to have to do a lot of relaxation exercises or meditation to keep your cool, because it's not something you can force your child to accept until he or she finds it on his/her own.

Conflict with your child can be stressful, and we encourage you to look for support from your peers — the many thousands of parents who've come before you. Finding a support group for parents online is easy—simply do a search on "support groups parents diabetes" and a number of results will pop up. One of the most popular groups is available through the web site www.childrenwithdiabetes.org, but there are others available through social networking sites such as www.tudiabetes.org, www.diabeticrockstar.com, and others. Parents can also find one-on-one support through the JDRF's online diabetes support team, which is staffed by volunteers who have "been there" with their own children. Some clinics that treat children with Type 1 diabetes also have their own online resources as well.

If you don't have access to a computer, finding a support group where members meet on a regular basis can be a bit more challenging, particularly if you live in a rural area far from a large town or city. Your best bet is to contact the American Diabetes Association by phone at 1-800-DIABETES (1-800-342-2383) and ask them to mail you information regarding diabetes support groups in your area (be sure to specify that you want groups for parents of children with Type 1 diabetes). The ADA's hours of operation are Monday–Friday, 8:30 AM–8 PM Eastern Standard Time. Alternatively, you might ask the clinic or hospital where your child is being treated whether they have (or would be willing to start) a support group for parents of children with diabetes.

100. Where can I go for more information?

There are many places with information about Type 1 diabetes. A search online using the keyword "Type 1 diabetes" will undoubtedly find thousands, if not tens of thousands, of sources of information—not all of it useful or relevant, and some of it flat out incorrect. The resources we offer in the Appendix are what we consider the best, most accurate we've found, and they're a good starting point for finding more information.

ADVOCACY ORGANIZATIONS

American Diabetes Association

The ADA's mission is to prevent and cure diabetes and to improve the lives of all people affected by diabetes. ADA funds research to prevent, cure and manage diabetes, delivers services to hundreds of communities, provides objective and credible information, and works on behalf of individuals denied their rights because of diabetes. The web site has a wealth of information and is particularly useful in relation to finding information about legal protections for children with diabetes, 504 Plans, and healthcare coverage. The ADA also offers an "Everyday Wisdom Kit" containing resources on caring for children with diabetes. This kit is available to parents of newly diagnosed children at http://www.diabetes.org/living-with-diabetes/parents-and-kids/everyday-wisdom-kit.html, or by calling the ADA's 800 number (below).

American Diabetes Association

ATTN: National Call Center
1701 North Beauregard Street
Alexandria, Virginia 22311
Phone: 800-DIABETES (800-342-2383)
E-mail: AskADA@diabetes.org
Web site: www.diabetes.org

Children With Diabetes Foundation

The mission of the Children with Diabetes Foundation is to fund human clinical trials leading to cure and prevention of Type 1 diabetes. CWDF describes itself as "the venture capitalists of diabetes research, getting new, clinically relevant, innovative research off the ground."

Children With Diabetes Foundation
685 East Wiggins Street
Superior, Colorado 80027
E-mail: info@CWDFoundation.org
Web site: www.cwdfoundation.org

CWDF has two sub-branches, one that offers assistance in getting supplies for children with diabetes and another that works on educational issues facing children with diabetes. Info pertaining to these branches is available in the Diabetes Supplies — Assistance and Education sections that follow.

Diabetes Hands Foundation
The Diabetes Hands Foundation was created to offer support, information, and community for people with diabetes. They focus on developing online communities and grassroots political action in support of people with diabetes.

Diabetes Hands Foundation
Post Office Box 9421
Berkeley, California 94709
Phone: 650-283-4862
E-mail: info@diabeteshf.org.
Web site: http://diabeteshandsfoundation.org

Juvenile Diabetes Research Foundation International (JDRF)
JDRF is the worldwide leader for research to cure Type 1 diabetes. It sets the global agenda for diabetes research and is the largest charitable funder and advocate of

diabetes science worldwide. The mission of JDRF is to find a cure for diabetes and its complications through the support of research.

Juvenile Diabetes Research Foundation International
26 Broadway
New York, New York 10004
Phone: 800-533-CURE (2873)
E-mail: info@jdrf.org
Web site: www.jdrf.org

BOOKS ON HOW TO PARENT A CHILD WITH DIABETES AND HOW TO MANAGE DIABETES IN GENERAL

Besser, R. (2009). *Diabetes Through the Looking Glass: Seeing Diabetes from Your Child's Perspective.* London: Class Publishing.

Greenberg, R. (2009). *50 Diabetes Myths That Can Ruin Your Life and the 50 Diabetes Truths That Can Save It.* Cambridge, MA: Da Capo/Lifelong Books.

Loy, S., and Loy, B. (2007). *Getting a Grip on Diabetes: Quick Tips & Techniques for Kids and Teens.* Alexandria, VA: American Diabetes Association.

McCarthy, M. (2007). *The Everything Parent's Guide to Children with Juvenile Diabetes.* Avon, MA: Adams Media.

Rubin, A.L. (2004). *Type 1 Diabetes for Dummies.* Indianapolis, IN: Wiley Publishing, Inc.

Ruhl, J. (2008). *Blood Sugar 101: What They Don't Tell You About Diabetes.* Turners Falls, MA: Technion Books. (Note that this book was written for people with Type 2 diabetes, but it contains a great deal of information on blood sugar and complications that will be useful to parents of newly diagnosed children with Type 1 diabetes.)

Scheiner, G. (2004). *Think Like a Pancreas: A Practical Guide to Managing Diabetes with Insulin*. Cambridge, MA: Da Capo Press.

Walsh, J., and Roberts, R. (2006). *Pumping Insulin*, 4th Edition. San Diego: Torrey Pines Press.

BOOKS FOR EXPLAINING DIABETES TO CHILDREN

Gosselin, K., Freedman, M. (2004). *Taking Diabetes to School*. JayJo Books. (ages 4–8)

Lang, R., Huss, S. (2004). *Lara Takes Charge*. HLPI Books. (ages 9–12)

Loy, B., and Loy, S. (2004). *487 Really Cool Tips for Kids with Diabetes*. American Diabetes Association. (young adult)

Olson, M. (2003). *How I Feel: A Book About Diabetes*. Lantern Books. (ages 9–12)

CARB COUNTING RESOURCES

Diabetes Network has an excellent resource for educating yourself about carbohydrates and carb-counting. It can be found online at http://www.diabetesnet.com/diabetes_food_diet/carb_counting.php.

A more concise but still comprehensive discussion of carb counting can be found at the **University of Pittsburgh's** patient education site: http://www.upmc.com/healthatoz/patienteducation/documents/basiccarbcounting.pdf

CalorieKing offers specific carbohydrate values of different foods at http://www.calorieking.com. CalorieKing also puts out an annual food guide that is widely available in bookstores. The most recent edition is *2010 CalorieKing Calorie, Fat and Carbohydrate Counter*. These small, inexpensive guides are a must if you eat out a lot, as they contain the carb counts of many common restaurant chain offerings and other common foods.

CELIAC DISEASE AND GLUTEN-FREE LIVING

Celiac Disease Foundation

CDF is a non-profit, public benefit corporation dedicated to providing services and support regarding Celiac Disease and Dermatitis Herpetiformis, through programs of awareness, education, advocacy and research.

Celiac Disease Foundation

13251 Ventura Blvd. #1
Studio City, California 91604
Phone: (818) 990-2354
E-mail: cdf@celiac.org
Web site: http://www.celiac.org

A variety of web sites exists to offer tips, recipes, and support for gluten-free living for people with celiac disease. Some of these include:

www.celiac.com
www.glutino.com
www.glutenfreeliving.com
http://glutenfreemommy.com
www.livingwithout.com

CLINICAL TRIALS AND RESEARCH INFO

TrialNet Recruitment

To participate in the screening phase of the Natural History Study, you must be: (1) 1 to 45 years of age and have a brother, sister, child, or parent with Type 1 diabetes,

OR (2) 1 to 20 years of age and have a cousin, aunt, uncle, niece, nephew, half-sibling, or grandparent with Type 1 diabetes. In general, Type 1 diabetes is assumed if it developed before age 40 and required insulin injections within a year of diagnosis.

Phone: 800-HALT-DM1

Phone: 800-425-8361

Web site: www.diabetestrialnet.org

Other sources of clinical trial information related to Type 1 diabetes can be found at the JDRF's web site: http://www.jdrf.org/index.cfm?page_id=101984

DIABETES SUPPLIES—ASSISTANCE

Supplies For Children With Diabetes Foundation

The mission of SCWDF is to provide short-term diabetes supplies for children with Type 1 diabetes who are in emergency situations in which their families are unable to obtain the basic supplies for diabetes care. An emergency situation might be defined as loss of health insurance, loss of a parent's job, or a local disaster, combined with the family having no other resources with which to purchase diabetes supplies.

Web site: http://www.cwdfoundation.org/Supplies.htm

E-mail: anbond@comcast.net

Other sources of support for the cost of insulin, syringes, and diabetes supplies

There are pharmaceutical assistance programs offered directly by some drug companies for people with Type 1 diabetes who have little or no insurance to help offset the cost of supplies or prescription medications. **The Pharmaceutical Research and Manufacturers Association** (www.phrma.org) (800-762-4636) has information on such programs. If you don't have a computer, call 800-762-4636. **The Partnership for Prescription Assistance** (www.pparx.org) can connect you with hundreds of assistance programs that have joined together to provide savings to the uninsured (Phone: 888-477-2669). The **Together Rx Access Card** (www.togetherrxaccess .com, 800-444-4106) offers 25% to 40% off brand-name prescription medications at pharmacies nationwide.

The makers of various blood glucose meters also offer discounts and freebies to people with diabetes who don't have insurance coverage. Abbott Labs, makers of the Freestyle blood glucose meter, offers a discount card to people who do not have insurance coverage for test strips, and the meter itself is often available for free from various sources. Likewise, the OneTouch UltraMini meter can be obtained at no charge from the manufacturer. Sites intended to serve people with diabetes also frequently give away meters as well. Do an internet search on "free glucose meter" and you'll get a number of sites that explain the available products and costs, if any.

EDUCATION

504 Plans for children with diabetes

The **American Diabetes Association** web site includes a detailed section on what a 504 plan is, how to obtain one, and sample plans to use as a guide for creating your child's plan. Go to www.diabetes.org and search on "504 Plan" to find this information.

You can also find their booklet on advocating for your child in the school system online: http://www.diabetes .org/assets/pdfs/schools/becomingdiabetesadvocate-schools.pdf

The **National Dissemination Center for Children with Disabilities** provides information to the nation on disabilities in children and youth; programs and services for infants, children, and youth with disabilities; IDEA, the nation's special education law; No Child Left Behind, the nation's general education law; and research-based information on effective practices for children with disabilities. Services are for families, educators, administrators, journalists, and students. The organization's special focus is children and youth (birth to age 22).

NICHCY
1825 Connecticut Avenue NW, Suite 700
Washington, DC 20009
Phone: (800) 695-0285
Fax: (202) 884-8441
E-mail: nichcy@aed.org
Web site: www.nichcy.org

One of the most useful pages the web site offers is a page that organizes all relevant educational contact information by state: www.nichcy.org/Pages/StateSpecificInfo .aspx

The **Disability Rights Education & Defense Fund** provides information for parents of children with disabilities who have experienced discrimination or educational neglect in their schools or community. The Fund has staff attorneys available for free legal advocacy support through their web site, by phone, or by e-mail.

2212 Sixth Street
Berkeley, California 94710
Toll-free: 800-348-4232 (v/tty)
Phone: 510-644-2555 (v/tty)
Fax: 510-841-8645

E-mail: info@dredf.org
Web site: www.dredf.org

More information about disability and anti-discrimination laws is available on the **Children With Diabetes** web site, http://www.childrenwithdiabetes.com/d_0q_600.htm

FINANCIAL HELP

National Diabetes Information Clearinghouse
National Institute of Diabetes and Digestive and Kidney Diseases (NIDDK)

Financial Help for Diabetes Care resource page:
http://diabetes.niddk.nih.gov/dm/pubs/financialhelp/

GLYCEMIC INDEX

The **Glycemic Index Foundation** (www.gifoundation.com) offers explanations of glycemic index and glycemic load.

NutritionData (http://www.nutritiondata.com/topics/glycemic-index) discusses glycemic index and glycemic load and offers lists comparing the glycemic indices of various foods.

HEALTH INSURANCE FOR CHILDREN WITH DIABETES

Every state in the nation has a health insurance program for infants, children, and teens who are not otherwise insured. To find out about programs in your state, search **Insure Kids Now!** (www.insurekidsnow.gov), offered by the **U.S. Department of Health & Human Services** (or call 877-KIDS-NOW).

Another option to investigate is your state **Children's Health Insurance Program** (www.cms.hhs.gov/home/chip.asp). Also, the **National Institute of Diabetes and Digestive and Kidney Diseases** (www.niddk.nih.gov) has a publication entitled "Financial Help for Diabetes Care." Order print copies from the National Diabetes Information Clearinghouse by calling 800-860-8747, or view it on the web at: http://diabetes.niddk.nih.gov/dm/pubs/financialhelp/

ONLINE COMMUNITY AND SUPPORT RESOURCES

www.childrenwithdiabetes.com

This site offers an online informational and community resource focused on children with diabetes and their parents. The site offers a family support network that includes chat rooms, information on schools and camps, a service that connects parents of young children with babysitters who understand Type 1 diabetes care, and links to a wide range of state-specific resources for parents.

www.tudiabetes.org

An online community for individuals with diabetes and the people who love them; includes discussion groups for children with diabetes, parents of children with diabetes, parents of toddlers with diabetes, insulin pump users, and a multitude of other categories. It is a highly recommended resource for parents of newly diagnosed children, as well as for the children themselves. The sister site, www.estudiabetes.org, provides the same services in Spanish.

www.diabeticrockstar.org

An online community for individuals with diabetes. Similar in goals to tudiabetes.org, it focuses more on supporting an attitude of self-sufficiency and high self-esteem among its members. It is a great resource for adolescents and young adults.

www.insulin-pumpers.org

An online community focused on providing information and support for people with diabetes who are using or considering insulin pump therapy.

www.isletsofhope.com

A diabetes support organization that contains comprehensive resources for people with diabetes.

504 Plan A plan created with school officials that spells out what accommodations the school will make to manage the special needs of a child with a legal disability, such as diabetes.

A

Activity profile The timing of a form of insulin's activity levels, including its peak activity and duration.

Artificial pancreas A mechanical device, still in development, that combines insulin pump, CGM technology, and other features to function much like a real pancreas.

Autoantibodies Antibodies that trigger immune cell attacks against the body's own cells.

Autoimmune disorder A disorder in which the immune system mistakenly attacks the body's own cells as if they were pathogens.

B

Basal insulin The low, constant level of insulin that is always present in the bloodstream.

Beta cells Cells within the pancreas that secrete insulin. In type 1 diabetes, beta cells are attacked and destroyed by an autoimmune response.

Blood glucose (also **blood sugar**) Concentration of glucose circulating in the bloodstream at any given time. Blood glucose is not constant, but changes depending on the food you eat, the time of day, the amount of exercise you get, and other factors.

Blood glucose meter A mechanical device that uses a drop of blood to assess current blood glucose levels.

Bolus A dose of insulin given all at once in response to food intake, or to correct a high blood sugar.

C

Cannula A very fine plastic tube inserted under the skin to deliver insulin.

Carb ratios The amount of insulin used for each gram of carbohydrate eaten.

Carbohydrates Compounds in food that are broken down into glucose. Carbohydrates can be simple (for example, sugar or fruit juice) or complex (whole grains).

Celiac disease An autoimmune response in the gut triggered by a protein found in wheat, rye, and barley. People with Type 1 diabetes have an increased risk of developing celiac disease.

Continuous glucose monitor (CGM) A mechanical device that monitors blood glucose levels and issues a warning when levels fall below or climb above the ideal range.

Co-occur A disease that occurs in tandem with or at the same time as another disease.

Correction factor A measurement of insulin sensitivity used to calculate the amount of insulin needed to correct a specific proportion of blood glucose above the upper limit of the acceptable range.

Correction scale The series of correction doses in relation to specific ranges of high blood sugar measurements.

Crash A sudden onset of hypoglycemic symptoms related to a rapid drop in blood glucose levels to hypoglycemic values, either because of high activity levels or too much insulin.

D

Dawn phenomenon High blood sugars that occur in the morning. In children, especially adolescents, these episodes are usually a result of the patterns of growth hormone secretion, which in adolescents tends to be most active from 3 AM to 10 AM.

Diabetes insipidus A form of diabetes related to the inability to concentrate urine. It is unrelated to diabetes mellitus.

Diabetes mellitus Any form of diabetes in which the interaction of insulin and blood glucose has become impaired.

Diabetic ketoacidosis (DKA) A complication of diabetes that occurs when ketones build up in the bloodstream sufficiently to lower blood pH below its normal level of about 7.35. DKA can be life threatening if untreated.

E

Endocrinologist A doctor specializing in hormonal disorders.

G

Genetic predisposition Having a gene or set of genes that makes one more likely to get a specific disease.

Glucagon A pancreatic hormone that stops insulin from transferring glucose into the cells.

Glucagon kit A pre-loaded emergency kit used to treat extreme low blood sugars containing a syringe, saline, and powdered glucagon.

Glucose A simple sugar derived from carbohydrate foods that the body's cells use for energy.

Gluten A protein found in grains such as wheat, rye, and barley that can trigger an autoimmune response in the digestive tract called celiac disease.

Glycemic index A measure of the rate at which certain foods cause blood glucose to rise.

Glycemic load A way of measuring how much and how fast a given portion of food will raise blood sugar.

Glycogen Glucose that has been stored in the liver. Glycogen is converted back into glucose and released into the bloodstream if blood glucose levels fall too low.

Glycohemoglobin Hemoglobin to which glucose is bound; a measure of long-term control of diabetes mellitus. Also called **glycosylated hemoglobin**.

H

Hemoglobin A protein in blood that carries oxygen to the cells.

Hemoglobin A1c test A blood test measuring the amount of glycosylated hemoglobin in the blood; the test gives a good indication of how well blood glucose is controlled over a 3-month time span.

Honeymoon A period of time post-diagnosis when beta cells in the pancreas resume producing some insulin.

Hormone Chemicals released from gland cells that signal to other cells to perform certain functions or actions. Insulin, for example, signals to cells that they should allow glucose to pass through the cell membrane.

Hyperglycemia High blood glucose levels.

Hypoglycemia Low blood glucose levels.

I

Immune system The collection of cells and actions that the body uses to fight off diseases, injuries, and toxic substances.

Infusion set The clip and tubing that connects the insulin reservoir of an insulin pump to the insertion site where the cannula has been inserted under the skin.

Infusion site The needle, adhesive, port, and cannula combination that is used to infuse insulin under the skin when using an insulin pump.

Insulin A hormone secreted by beta cells in the pancreas. Insulin is responsible for transporting glucose from the bloodstream into cells for energy.

Insulin pump A mechanical device that gives basal and bolus doses of insulin as programmed by the pump user via a cannula inserted under the skin.

Insulin resistance Loss of a cell's ability to respond to insulin appropriately.

Intermediate-acting insulin Insulin that has been synthesized to have an 8- to 12-hour activity profile.

K

Ketoacidosis A condition of low blood pH because of the presence of ketones in the blood. In people with diabetes, ketoacidosis generally occurs when a person has too little insulin for too long.

Ketogenesis Production of ketones.

Ketone bodies See **ketones**.

Ketones Acidic by-products of fat burning that can be harmful if generated for long periods of time.

L

Lidocaine A common numbing cream used to desensitize skin before inserting an insulin pump cannula.

Long-acting insulin Insulin that has been synthesized to have a 24-hour activity profile.

M

Manually delivered insulin (MDI) Insulin delivered by means of a syringe.

Metabolic disorder A malfunction in the body's usual means of transporting and transforming food, water, and air into molecules that cells can use to live, function, and reproduce.

Multiple daily injections (MDI) The treatment protocol in which insulin is manually delivered using syringes.

P

Pancreas A gland of the digestive system that is responsible for releasing insulin, glucagon, digestive enzymes, and other hormones. The inability of the pancreas to produce insulin is the key problem in type 1 diabetes.

Pediatric endocrinologist A doctor specializing in hormonal disorders in children. Because children are growing, their hormones and metabolic needs differ from those of adults.

R

Rapid-acting insulin Insulin that begins to act within 15 minutes and generally lasts about 4 hours, peaking within 2-3 hours.

Retinopathy Damage to the eye that distorts the retina and leads to vision loss in people with diabetes.

S

Short-acting insulin Insulin that begins to work within an hour and lasts about 4 hours.

Stacking Overlapping doses of insulin that cause low blood sugar levels.

Subcutaneous Below the skin.

T

Target range The range of blood glucose values considered acceptable in a child with diabetes. The target range varies according to age and time of day.

Trigger An event that activates a genetic predisposition for autoimmunity, such as a viral infection or an exposure to toxic chemicals.

Type 2 diabetes A common form of diabetes mellitus that occurs mostly in adults and is caused by the inability of cells to respond to insulin.

Index